EXERCISES FOR
DIABETES

Simple Steps for Better Health

By Erin O'Driscoll, R.N., M.A.

Photography by Peter Field Peck

healthyliving**books**

New York • London

Text © 2005 Erin O'Driscoll
Photographs © 2005 Hatherleigh Press, Inc.

A Healthy Living Book
Hatherleigh Press
5–22 46th Avenue, Suite 200
Long Island City, NY 11101
www.healthylivingbooks.com

Library of Congress Cataloging-in-Publication Data

O'Driscoll, Erin.
  Exercise for diabetes / Erin O'Driscoll.
      p. cm.
  Includes bibliographical references.
  ISBN 1-57826-188-0
  1. Diabetes—Exercise therapy. I. Title.
  RC661.E94O38 2005
  616.4'62062—dc22
                            2005001936

Names of medications are typically followed by ® symbols, but these symbols are not stated in this book.

Brand names included in this book are provided as examples only, and their inclusion does not imply an endorsement. Also, if a particular brand name is not mentioned, this does not mean or imply that the product is unsatisfactory.

All forms of exercise pose some inherent risks. The information in this book is meant to supplement, not replace, proper exercise training. Before practicing the exercises in this book, be sure that your equipment is well maintained. Do not take risks beyond your level of experience, training, and fitness. The exercise and dietary programs in this book are not intended as a substitute for any exercise routine or treatment or dietary regimen that may have been prescribed by your doctor. As with all exercise and dietary programs, you should get your doctor's approval before beginning. The author(s), editors, and publisher advice readers to take full responsibility for their safety and know their limits.

Healthy Living Books titles are available for bulk purchase, special promotions, and premiums. For information about reselling and special purchase opportunities, please call 1-800-528-2550 and ask for the Special Sales Manager.

Cover and Interior Design by Deborah Miller and Phillip Mondestin
Photography by Peter Field Peck

10 9 8 7 6 5 4 3 2 1
Printed in Canada

Table of Contents

Introduction iv

Part I: About Diabetes v

  Chapter 1: The Face of Diabetes: The New Epidemic? 1

  Chapter 2: What is Diabetes? 4

  Chapter 3: Types of Diabetes 8

  Chapter 4: The Importance of Managing Your Diabetes 14

  Chapter 5: Complications 28

  Chapter 6: Diet and Weight Control 40

  Chapter 7: Benefits of Exercise for Diabetics 55

Part II: Exercises for Diabetes 59

  Chapter 8: Exercise Recommendations for Diabetics 61

  Chapter 9: Aerobics Exercises 75

  Chapter 10: Strength Exercises 106

  Chapter 11: Flexibility Training, Warm Ups, and Cool-Downs 127

Part III: The Workouts 153

  Chapter 12: The Mini-Trampoline Aerobics Program 155

  Chapter 13: The Floor Aerobics Program .165

  Chapter 14: The Strength-Training Program 173

  Chapter 15: Fitness Walking 176

  Chapter 16: Cycling 179

Appendix A: Training Log 181

Appendix B: Websites 183

Appendix C: References 184

Introduction

Approximately 11 million Americans have diabetes mellitus. Complications of this disease make it the third leading cause of death in America. It is time for a wake-up call.

Exercise is particularly important in managing or even preventing diabetes. Most people with diabetes are encouraged to participate in a regular program of exercise, but must be careful when starting an exercise program because of its effects on the body's glucose. The purpose of this book is to educate you on managing your diabetes and to give suggestions on how to lead an active lifestyle.

Exercise and modification of your diet are the cornerstones in the management of diabetes. Exercise alone is very important in controlling glucose levels and reducing the risk factors of heart disease. Early identification and treatment of diabetes can help you control your diabetes and can allow you to live a longer and healthier life. Diabetes, unfortunately, is one of the risk factors for the development of heart disease. A sedentary couch potato lifestyle is also a risk factor, which is why exercise is so important. Why have two strikes against you? Exercise does make a difference and this book will guide you on how to exercise safely and effectively with diabetes mellitus.

Part I: About Diabetes

1

The Face of Diabetes: The New Epidemic?

Each day approximately 2,200 people are diagnosed with diabetes. This chronic disease has no cure, and the costs associated with managing diabetes are estimated at 91.8 billion dollars per year. A diabetic will spend an average of $13,242 on medical expenses, for example, and someone without the disease will spend only $2,560. Over 80 percent of diabetics die from a heart or blood vessel disease, and according to the Society for Women's Health Research, a diabetic woman's risk of heart attack is more than twice that of a non-diabetic woman.

If you are overweight or bordering on obesity, you have a greater risk of developing type 2 diabetes. In fact, 80 percent of type 2 diabetics are overweight. Unfortunately, type 2 diabetes, once believed to occur primarily in adulthood, is now being diagnosed in children and teenagers with greater frequency. Currently about 25 percent of new type 2 diabetes cases are diagnosed in teenagers. The rise of obesity in children, due largely to junk-food diets and inadequate activity, may be the greatest contributor to the development of diabetes. So, the primary goal for all age groups is weight reduction and fat loss. You can lower your body fat and increase your lean muscle with a combination of aerobic conditioning and strength training.

Type 2 diabetes is more common in older people, especially in people who are overweight, and occurs more often in African-Americans, Native Americans, some Asian-Americans, Native Hawaiians and other Pacific Islander Americans, and Hispanic-Americans. On average, non-Hispanic African-Americans are 1.6 times as likely to have diabetes as non-Hispanic whites of the same age. Hispanic-Americans are 1.5 times as likely to have diabetes as non-Hispanic whites of similar age. Native Americans have one of the highest rates of diabetes in the world. On average, Native Americans and Native Alaskans are 2.3 times as likely to have diabetes as non-Hispanic whites of similar age.

About 206,000 people under 20 years of age have diabetes. As obesity rates in children continue to soar, type 2 diabetes, a disease that used to be seen primarily in adults over age 45, is becoming more common in young people. Diabetes presents unique issues for children and teens. Simple things—like going to a birthday party, playing sports, or staying overnight with friends—need careful planning. Children with diabetes may need to take insulin or oral medication every day. They also need to check their blood glucose several times during the day and remember to make correct food choices. These tasks can make school-age children feel "different" from their classmates. These tasks can be particularly bothersome for teens.

For any child or teen with diabetes, learning to cope with the disease is a big job. Dealing with a chronic illness such as diabetes may cause emotional and behavioral challenges. Talking to a social worker or psychologist may help young people and their families learn to adjust to lifestyle changes needed to stay healthy.

It is a sad fact that the Centers for Disease Control and Prevention (CDC) reported that 15 percent of 6- to 19-year-old Americans, nearly 9 million, are overweight. We hear about it all the time on television and in news articles. Increasing public awareness is a good start, but an effective way to reverse this trend is to educate children on proper nutrition and to encourage physical activity that is fun. Consequently, this may prevent the early onset of complications associated with diabetes. This book includes aerobic exercise using a mini-trampoline that can help burn calories and improve weight loss that kids and teens can enjoy too!

You may question the role of heredity in the development of diabetes in young people; however, it has been found that the increased numbers of cases of diabetes being diagnosed cannot be attributed to genetics alone. Lack of exercise and overeating are other culprits. Fortunately, this can be changed with exercise and a proper diet.

Males in particular are susceptible to developing diabetes due to the way they gain weight. Males tend to accumulate fat in the upper body, in particular the abdominal area, a pattern referred to as an apple shape. Females gain weight in a pear-shaped pattern—that is, in the lower body: on the hips, buttocks, and thighs. Research has shown that the apple shape is associated with a higher risk for developing diabetes and other diseases such as high blood pressure, coronary artery disease, and stroke.

The prevalence of diabetes in the United States is likely to increase for several reasons. First, a large segment of the population is aging. Also, Hispanic-Americans and other groups that tend to be susceptible to diabetes make up the fastest-growing segment of the U.S. population. Finally, Americans are increasingly overweight and sedentary. According to recent estimates, the prevalence of diabetes in the United States is predicted to reach 8.9 percent of the population by 2025. The rise in diabetes is being attributed to the rise in obesity.

2

What Is Diabetes?

Whether you have recently been diagnosed with diabetes or you have had diabetes for a while, look at the statistics and realize you are not alone. There are millions of others with the same struggles. It is time to educate yourself and keep your diabetes under control.

To understand diabetes you need to know the two major players: blood glucose and insulin. When you have diabetes, your body either does not produce or does not properly use insulin. Normally, the body breaks down food (especially carbohydrates) into sugar or glucose. Glucose is transported through the bloodstream to be used as an energy source. Insulin, a hormone, is secreted by the beta cells of the pancreas. It transports glucose into the muscle cells where it is converted and used as energy. Insulin helps to regulate blood sugar levels and keep them within the normal range. You should always have a certain amount of glucose in the bloodstream to be available when you need it.

Having diabetes means that your blood glucose (often called blood sugar) is too high. Glucose comes from the foods you eat and is also made in your liver and muscles. Your blood carries the glucose to all the cells in your body and then insulin helps the glucose from food travel to your cells. If your body doesn't make enough insulin or if the insulin doesn't work the way it should, glucose isn't able to get into your cells and stays in your blood instead. Your blood glucose levels then get too high, causing pre-diabetes or diabetes. Your blood always has some glucose in it because your body needs glucose for energy to keep you going, but too much glucose in the blood isn't good for your health. Controlling your diabetes means managing blood glucose levels through diet, exercise, and medications that your doctor may prescribe.

Many people have no signs or symptoms. Symptoms can also be so mild that you might not even notice them. Nearly six million people in the United States have type 2 diabetes and do not know it. Here is what to look for:

- increased thirst
- increased hunger
- fatigue
- increased urination, especially at night
- weight loss
- blurred vision
- sores that do not heal

You may have had one or more of these signs before you found out you had diabetes. Or you may have had no signs at all. A blood test to check your glucose levels will show if you have diabetes.

Sometimes people have symptoms but do not suspect diabetes. They delay scheduling a checkup because they do not feel sick. Many people do not find out they have the disease until they have diabetes complications, such as blurry vision or heart trouble. It is important to find out early if you have diabetes because treatment can prevent damage to the body from diabetes.

Anyone 45 years old or older should consider getting tested for diabetes. If you are 45 or older and overweight, it is strongly recommended that you get tested. If you are younger than 45, overweight, and have one or more of the risk factors below, you should consider testing. Ask your doctor for a fasting blood glucose test or an oral glucose tolerance test. Your doctor will tell you if you have diabetes.

As mentioned in Chapter 1, type 2 diabetes is more common in the elderly, especially in the overweight, and occurs more often in African-Americans, American Indians, some Asian-Americans, Native Hawaiians and other Pacific Islander Americans, and Hispanic-Americans. Here are other risk factors for diabetes:

- Age—45 and older
- Overweight—body mass index greater than or equal to 25 (23 if Asian-American, 26 if Pacific Islander)
- Ethnicity—African-American, Native American, Asian-American, Hispanic-American and Latino American, or Pacific Islander heritage
- Family history—have a first-degree relative with diabetes
- History of gestational diabetes or giving birth to a baby weighing more than 9 pounds
- Hypertension—blood pressure greater than 140/90
- Abnormal lipid levels—HDL cholesterol level less than 40 mg/dl for men and less than 50 mg/dl for women; triglyceride level greater than 250 mg/dl
- IGT or IFG on previous testing
- Polycystic ovary syndrome or acanthosis nigricans
- History of vascular disease
- Inactive lifestyle—exercise less than three times a week

Even if you have any of these risk factors, much can be done to lower your chances of getting diabetes. Exercising regularly, reducing fat and calorie intake, and losing weight can all help you reduce your risk of developing type 2 diabetes. Lowering blood pressure and cholesterol levels also helps you stay healthy.

It is becoming clear that high blood pressure, coronary artery disease, obesity, and diabetes share a common pathway. There appears to be a very strong link between obesity and the development of diabetes. It is mind-boggling that 61 percent of American adults are overweight or obese and so are at risk of developing heart disease, diabetes, arthritis, and several forms of cancer. Research has shown that losing as little as 5 to 10 percent of body weight has significant effects in reducing the development of diabetes. Interestingly, in a study conducted on obese patients with diabetes that underwent gastric-bypass surgery, it was discovered that 78 percent experienced a reversal of their diabetic condition.

Obesity has been attributed to many factors, including hormonal imbalance, emotional disturbances, cultural habits, environmental influences, inadequate physical activity, and poor diet. Whatever the cause, obesity is a major player in the development of diabetes. With obesity, the beta cells (discussed earlier) of the pancreas often become less sensitive or responsive to high levels of glucose concentrations. The insulin in the blood is less effective in transporting glucose into the cell, because of the reduction in the number of insulin receptors on the muscle and other target cells in the body. It is also believed that some of these receptors for insulin become inactive with obesity.

To state it more simply, fat cells block the doorway, preventing glucose and its carrier insulin from crossing the threshold into the cell to be used as energy.

3

Types of Diabetes

There are two types of diabetes, type 1 and type 2. With type 1, your body makes little or no insulin. This type of diabetes is believed to be an autoimmune disease that first occurs most often in children and young adults. Type 1 diabetics must take daily injections of insulin to lower their blood glucose levels. Type 2 diabetes, or non-insulin dependent diabetes mellitus (NIDDM), is a metabolic disorder. The pancreas can produce insulin, but it may not be enough, or the body's cells have trouble using the insulin properly. That's because the body resists the insulin that helps the sugar move into the cells. Although some sugar is used, it is not enough.

Type 1 Diabetes

Type 1 diabetes, formerly called juvenile diabetes or insulin-dependent diabetes, is usually first diagnosed in children, teenagers, or young adults. In this form of diabetes, the beta cells of the pancreas no longer make insulin because the body's immune system has attacked and destroyed them. Type 1 diabetes may account for 5 to 10 percent of all diagnosed cases of diabetes. The risk factors for type 1 diabetes are less well-defined than those for type 2 diabetes (listed in Chapter 2). Autoimmune, genetic, and environmental factors are involved in developing this type of diabetes. Treatment for type 1 diabetes includes taking insulin shots or using an insulin pump, making wise food choices, exercising regularly, taking aspirin daily (for some), and controlling blood pressure and cholesterol.

Type 1 diabetes affects as many as 1 in 500 children. This number may be increasing because of the advancements made in therapies to manage the disease. More children are living longer and passing the genetic trait onto their own children. Children with type 1 diabetes must take insulin because the pancreas can not produce it. The age of onset is usually between 5 to 7 years or at puberty, and it can develop very suddenly, with significant weight loss being the first sign. Other symptoms are:

- thirst
- frequent urination
- fatigue
- blurred vision
- itching
- mood changes
- glucose in the urine

Children need to learn how to monitor their glucose levels just as adults do. Children should receive education and support regarding proper nutrition, exercise, and daily diabetic self-management.

In the past, children diagnosed with diabetes were assumed to have type 1 diabetes. However, the tide is turning. Before 1990, only

5 percent of children or adolescents diagnosed with diabetes were classified as having type 2. It is now estimated that 30 to 50 percent of all new cases of diabetes diagnosed in the young are type 2. It is no coincidence that these numbers coincide with the rise in adolescent and childhood obesity.

Just like adults, children are at risk of developing diabetes based on ethnic background, excess weight, family history, and insulin resistance. As mentioned earlier, insulin resistance occurs when the muscle, fat, and liver cells resist the insulin molecule on the cell membrane. Healthy food choices and exercise need to be a priority for diabetic children. Children need to watch less television, limit the playing of computer games, and increase their daily physical activity. There is no cure for diabetes but you can certainly prevent or delay its development. It has been demonstrated that people with prediabetes can reduce their risk of getting diabetes by up to 58 percent with only 30 minutes of daily exercise and a low-fat diet, which usually produces the desired weight loss.

So how do you get kids to be more active? You need to be a little creative. Fitness must be fun, or kids just won't do it. The trampoline exercises featured in this book are a great place to start. Kids love the trampoline! Think about setting up a fitness obstacle course in your yard or basement. Many household items can be incorporated into a fitness obstacle course. Here are a few ideas on how to set up your own obstacle course:

Stool: Have your child step up and down on the step (10x on the right leg, 10x on the left leg).

Bleach bottles: Fill bottles with water and place a line of masking tape at two points on the floor. The goal is to carry the bleach bottles from point A to point B.

Hula hoops: Arrange the hoops in an interesting pattern on the floor and direct your child to jump from hoop to hoop.

Crepe paper: Tape crepe paper strips across the room, or on the backs of chairs. Tape them at various levels so the child will need to crawl under some and jump over others.

Masking tape: Tape a line of tape on the floor, either in a straight line or at several angles. The child can walk the line and pretend it is a tight rope. This will also help develop balance.

Ball dribble: Have your child dribble a ball along the masking tape line. The goal is to stay as close to the line as possible.

Rope: Cut a length of fairly heavy rope in order to use it as a jump rope.

These are just a few suggestions to create a fitness obstacle course that will get your children and their friends up and moving. You can time them as they move through the course, or let them perform the exercises at their own pace. The fitness obstacle course works well at kid's parties. You can also add items that you can purchase, such as a mini-trampoline or a stationary cycle.

Type 2 Diabetes

Type 2 diabetes, formerly called adult-onset diabetes or noninsulin-dependent diabetes, is the most common form of diabetes. Type 2 diabetes may account for about 90 to 95 percent of all diagnosed cases of diabetes. People can develop type 2 diabetes at any age—even during childhood.

It appears that the driving force for the development of type 2 diabetes is insulin resistance. As insulin resistance develops, insulin-sensitive tissues become resistant to its actions. In particular, muscle and liver cells become less sensitive to insulin circulating in the bloodstream. The pancreas responds to the increased blood glucose levels by secreting more insulin in an attempt to normalize the blood glucose. Constant and prolonged elevated insulin levels exhaust the pancreas, causing it to stop producing insulin. Blood sugar runs wild and medication must be taken to control it. With either type 1 or type 2 diabetes, your blood sugar stays too high, a condition called hyperglycemia. Exercise enhances the removal of glucose from the bloodstream into the muscle cells. Over time this will lower blood glucose levels.

Adipose or fat tissue is a major contributor to insulin resistance. Because insulin resistance can be decreased when body fat is reduced, weight loss by exercise should be your major objective.

Treatment includes using diabetes medicines, making wise food choices, exercising regularly, taking aspirin daily, and controlling blood pressure and cholesterol.

Gestational Diabetes

During some pregancies, glucose levels become elevated in what is known as gestational diabetes. Approximately 2 to 3 percent of all women who did not have diabetes prior to becoming pregnant become diabetic during pregnancy. Gestational diabetes is not caused by a lack of insulin, but by insulin resistance. It usually is diganosed at midpoint of pregnancy when insulin resistance becomes most noticeable. The diabetic condition usually disappears after delivery, but the mother has an increased risk, as high as 50 to 60 percent, of developing type 2 diabetes later in life.

Risk factors for gestational diabetes include:
- obesity
- pregnancy when over 30 years of age
- history of large babies (over 10 lbs)
- history of unexplained miscarriage
- family history of diabetes
- history of congenital anomalies in previous pregnancies

All women should be screened for gestational diabetes during pregnancy. This is usually done with an oral glucose screening test at 24 to 28 weeks of pregnancy. If you are at high risk for the development of diabetes than you should be screened earlier. Gestational diabetes can usually be managed with diet. Exercise, insulin therapy, blood glucose monitoring, and fetal assessment tests also play an important role in the care of the diabetic pregnant women.

The unique concerns and circumstances of the pregnant diabetic are beyond the scope of this book. Children and pregnant women are special populations that respond differently physiologically to exercise and therefore have their own set of guidelines and recommendations. This book's focus is mainly on the young to middle-aged diabetic exerciser with type 2 diabetes.

4

The Importance of Managing Your Diabetes

Managing diabetes is largely a matter of monitoring and controlling your blood glucose, blood pressure, and cholesterol levels. These three numbers will tell you if you are at risk of developing heart disease, kidney disease, or other complications.

Know Your Blood Glucose Levels

Know your numbers. I cannot emphasize enough the importance of monitoring and controlling your blood glucose levels. It is quite a task, but you have to do it! Taking control of your diabetes will help you feel better and stay healthy. Diet, exercise, and medication are the most important ways to be in control. You'll need to know your blood sugar numbers to be sure you are managing your sugar levels effectively. The American Diabetes Association recommends that all diabetics routinely test their blood sugar levels.

There are two ways you can test your blood sugar. One way requires a simple lab test called a hemoglobin A1c test, also called the HBA one C or A1c test. This test gives you a picture of your blood sugar levels. If your level is higher than 8 percent, you will need to discuss with your doctor how to bring your numbers down. You should take this lab test at least twice a year.

A second method for testing is a blood sugar test you can do yourself using a drop of blood and a glucose meter. Testing your own blood sugar is the best measure for daily diabetes control. Self-testing, using a meter, helps you see how food, physical activities, and medications affect your blood sugar. There are many pocket-size, convenient, and easy-to-use meters on the market today. Your doctor will help you decide what your goal numbers should be. Basic blood sugar goals for most diabetics are: 80 to 120 mg/dl before meals and 100 to 140mg/dl before bedtime. You should test your blood sugar before meals, before and after exercise, and at bedtime. It seems like a lot but keeping your levels steady will keep you healthy and prevent possible eye, kidney, and nerve damage.

- Discuss your blood glucose target with your health ceare team and keep a record of it.
- Discuss what you need to do to reach your target.
- Ask if you need to test your blood glucose yourself, and how often.

Know Your Blood Pressure

High blood pressure, also known as hypertension, is a condition in which the blood vessels become narrow, causing an increase in pressure inside the vessels. You can compare your blood vessels to a garden hose. If you squeeze down a garden hose, you can feel the water pressure increase. The pressure rises because the water is forced through a smaller space. It is the same idea with blood vessels. When plaque forms on the inside of the vessels, it reduces the space where blood can flow. Over time, this increased pressure can damage your vessels.

Having diabetes increases your risk for developing high blood pressure. Controlling or preventing diabetes, along with a low-fat, low cholesterol diet to reduce plaque formation, will decrease your risk for developing hypertension.

Normal blood pressure is 120/80. Desireable blood pressure is even slightly lower. You have high blood pressure if your numbers are 140/90 or higher. If you have diabetes you are considered hypertensive wih a blood pressure reading of 130/85. Blood pressure can be controlled by certain medications such as ACE inhibitors, beta-blockers, calcium channel blockers, vasodilars, and diuretics. Exercise and weight loss can help too.

- Ask your health care team what your blood pressure is and keep a dated record of the results.
- Discuss your blood pressure target with your health care team and write it down.
- Discuss what you need to do to reach your target.
- Ask if you need to test your blood pressure yourself. If so, find out how and when, and what supplies you need.

Know Your Cholesterol

Your total cholesterol should be less than 200 mg/dl. You have two primary types of cholesterol: low density lipoproteins (LDL) which are considered "bad" cholesterol, and high density lipoproteins (HDL) or "good" cholesterol. Your LDL should be less than 130, or less than 100 for diabetics, and your HDL should be greater than 35. Exercise can help increase HDL cholesterol. In fact an HDL of greater than 60 can have a protective effect against heart attack. Your triglycerides (a third form of fat) should be less than 200.

Lowering your cholesterol will also reduce the health risks associated with diabetes. You can cut the fat and cholesterol in your diet by limiting fat to 25 to 35 percent of your total calories each day. Carbohydrates such as breads, cereals, rice, and grains should provide 50 to 60 percent of your calories. The other 15 percent should come from lean meats, skinless chicken and turkey, fish, eggs, or beans. Cut back on margarine and butter, and choose the types that are whipped. They are lower in fat than stick butter.

- Discuss your LDL cholesterol target with your health care team and keep a record of the results.
- Discuss what you need to do to reach your target.

The Metabolic Syndrome

In the past, hypertension, insulin resistance, and high cholesterol were treated separately. Recently the medical community began linking them and collectively referring to these conditions as metabolic syndrome. Treatment strategies involve reducing risk factors, maintaining normal blood pressure, cholesterol, lipids, and body fat, and preventing complications. Exercise has been proven to have a positive effect on all three of these conditions.

Medications

Diet and exercise are important ways of controlling your diabetes. Unfortunately, it may not be enough. After you have had type 2 diabetes for a few years, your body may stop making enough insulin. Then you will need to take diabetes medications. Your doctor may recommend oral medications (pills, tablets), insulin injections, or a combination of both. But you need to know that diabetes medicines can never take the place of healthy eating and exercise. Even if you take medications you should still exercise because of many other health benefits, and follow a meal plan designed by a registered dietician to help control your weight.

There are several types of medications that may be prescribed by your doctor to control your blood sugar levels. The different drug categories control blood sugar in different ways. Some act to slow down the release of sugar into the blood, others cause the pancreas to make more insulin, and some make your body more sensitive to the insulin you do make. There are six groups of oral diabetic medicines.

Thiazolidinediones

Thiazolidinediones (THIGH-ah-ZO-li-deen-DYE-owns) make your cells more sensitive to insulin by helping the body use its own insulin more effectively. These drugs decrease the amount of sugar made by the liver, so the insulin can move glucose from your blood into your cells for energy. Two thiazolidinediones on the market are pioglitazone (Actos) and rosiglitazone (Avandia). If you take pioglitazone or rosiglitazone, it is important for your healthcare provider to check your liver enzyme levels regularly. Call your doctor right away if you have any signs of liver disease (nausea, vomiting, stomach pain, lack of appetite, tiredness, yellowing of the skin or whites of the eyes, or dark-colored urine). Some people who took troglitazone, another thiazolidinedione, have had serious liver problems. Troglitazone is no longer available.

There are side effects to this type of diabetes medication, including weight gain, anemia, and swelling in your legs or ankles (edema).

Sulfonylureas

For these pills to work, your pancreas has to make some insulin. Sulfonylureas can make your blood glucose too low, a condition called hypoglycemia (HY-po-gly-SEE-mee-ah). These pills help your pancreas make more insulin, which lowers your blood glucose and helps your body to better use the insulin it makes.

Side effects of sulfonylureas include hypoglycemia, upset stomach, a skin rash or itching, and weight gain.

Biguanides

This type of medication decreases the amount of sugar made by the liver. The biguanide metformin lowers blood glucose by making sure your liver does not make too much glucose. It also lowers the amount of insulin in your body. People may experience weight loss when starting metformin. This weight loss can help control blood glucose. Metformin can also improve blood fat and cholesterol levels, which are often not normal in people with type 2 diabetes.

Possible side effects include weakness, fatigue, dizziness, and trouble breathing. Nausea, diarrhea, and other digestive symptoms may arise when starting metformin. These usually go away. The mouth may also have a metallic taste.

Alpha-Glucosidase inhibitors

There are now two alpha-glucosidase inhibitors: acarbose (AK-er-bose) and miglitol (MIG-leh-tall). Both medicines block the enzymes that digest the starches you eat. This action causes a slower and lower rise of blood glucose through the day, but mainly right after meals. This drug acts on the intestines to slow the absorption of starches and sugars. Taking this pill may cause digestive problems (gas, bloating, and diarrhea) that most often go away after you take the medicine for a while.

Meglitinides

Meglitinides (meh-GLIT-in-ides) are another type of diabetes medicine. Repaglinide (re-PAG-lyn-ide) is the name of a meglitinide. This medicine helps your pancreas make more insulin right after meals, which is when you need it, leading to lower blood glucose levels. A good thing about repaglinide is that it works fast and your body uses it quickly. This fast action means you can vary the times you eat and the number of meals you eat more easily using repaglinide than you can using other diabetes medicines. Possible side effects of repaglinide include hypoglycemia and weight gain.

D-Phenylalanine Derivatives

Nateglinide (nah-TAG-lin-ide) is the first medicine in a new group of diabetes pills called D-phenylalanine (dee-fen-nel-AL-ah-neen) derivatives. Nateglinide helps your pancreas make more insulin quickly and for a short time. Then the insulin helps lower your blood glucose after you eat a meal.

This medicine may cause your blood glucose to drop too low. If you have liver disease, talk with your health care provider, since this medicine has not been tested in people with liver disease. Also, ask whether your other medicines might interact with nateglinide.

You may need only one type of medication or you may need to take several medications. Your doctor will recommend the therapy or combination of therapies that works best to control your blood sugar levels. You should always follow your doctor's recommendations regarding the dose, frequency, and timing of your medication. Always communicate with your doctor if you experience any side effects or if the medication is not doing its job. Your medication regime may change. Over time, most type 2 diabetics produce less and less insulin. Exercise and physical activity of varying intensities will also affect the way your body uses glucose. Therefore your treatment will probably change, too. You may need to start taking insulin as well.

Insulin

If your pancreas no longer makes enough insulin, you need to take insulin as a shot. Because insulin is a protein, if you took it orally, your body would break it down and digest it before it got into your blood to lower your blood glucose. Insulin lowers your blood glucose by moving glucose from your blood into the cells of your body. Once inside the cells, glucose provides energy. Insulin lowers your blood glucose whether you eat or not, and because of this you should eat on time if you are taking insulin. Possible side effects of insulin include hypoglycemia and weight gain.

There are six main types of insulin. They each work at different speeds. Many people take two types of insulin. The six types of insulin are:

RAPID-ACTING
>   insulin lispro (Humalog)
>>   Starts working in 5 to 15 minutes.
>>   Lowers blood glucose most in 45 to 90 minutes.
>>   Finishes working in 3 to 4 hours.
>   insulin aspart (Novolog)
>>   Starts working in 10 to 20 minutes.
>>   Lowers blood glucose most in 1 to 3 hours.
>>   Finishes working in 3 to 5 hours.

SHORT-ACTING
Regular (R) insulin
>>Starts working in 30 minutes.
>>Lowers blood glucose most in 2 to 5 hours.
>>Finishes working in 5 to 8 hours.

INTERMEDIATE-ACTING
NPH (N) or Lente (L) insulin
>>Starts working in 1 to 3 hours.
>>Lowers blood glucose most in 6 to 12 hours.
>>Finishes working in 16 to 24 hours.

LONG-ACTING
Ultralente (U) insulin
>>Starts working in 4 to 6 hours.
>>Lowers blood glucose most in 8 to 20 hours.
>>Finishes working in 24 to 28 hours.

VERY LONG-ACTING
insulin glargine (Lantus)
>>Starts working in 1 hour.
>>Lowers blood glucose evenly for 24 hours.
>>Finishes working in 24 hours and is taken once a day at bedtime.
>>Lantus should not be mixed together in a syringe with any other form of insulin before use.

PREMIXED
NPH and Regular insulin mixture
>>Two types of insulins mixed together in one bottle.
>>Starts working in 30 minutes.
>>Lowers blood sugar most in 7 to 12 hours.
>>Finishes working in 16 to 24 hours.

Injecting Insulin

Insulin should be injected just under the skin with a fine, short needle. Needle gauges available include 28g, 29g, 30g. (The higher the gauge the thinner the needle.) Needle lengths are 1/2" and 5/16".

With a shorter needle, you are less likely to inject insulin into your muscle. Injecting into a muscle can be more painful and lead to erratic blood glucose control. The depth of subcutaneous (below the skin) injection can affect the rate and amount of insulin absorption. Injecting into the muscle results in quicker insulin absorption, which can lead to hypoglycemia.

Sites for Insulin Injection

- Upper arm, front and outer thigh, buttock, and abdomen
- Avoid a 2" radius around the navel
- Rotate injection sites to prevent lipohypertrophy, the accumulation of fatty tissue, and to prevent lipoatrophy, small depressions in the subcutaneous tissue
- Different injection sites have different rates of absorption, which can produce erratic glucose levels.
- Choose a site according to the rate of absorption that may be needed at a given time. (Example: If you have a glucose level of 220mg/dl and plan to take your usual dose of rapid-acting insulin before eating, inject the insulin in the abdomen. If your glucose level is 78mg/dl, choose a site that has a slower rate of absorption, such as the thigh.)

Since exercise increases blood flow to the exercising muscle, injecting insulin into the working muscles of the extremities will increase the rate at which insulin is absorbed. You should inject the insulin into your abdomen rather than your arms or legs on the days that you exercise.

For safety reasons, needles should be disposed of in a hard plastic or metal container with a screw-on or tightly secured lid, such as a plastic bleach bottle or coffee can.

Alternative Medicine

The National Center for Complementary and Alternative Medicine, part of the National Institutes of Health, defines complementary and alternative medicine as a "group of diverse medical and health care systems, practices, and products that are not presently considered to be part of conventional medicine." Complementary medicine is used with conventional therapy, whereas alternative medicine is used instead of conventional medicine.

Some people with diabetes use complementary or alternative therapies to treat diabetes. Although some of these therapies may be effective, others can be ineffective or even harmful. Patients who use complementary and alternative medicine need to let their health care providers know what they are doing. Some complementary and alternative medicine therapies are discussed below. For more information, talk with your health-care provider.

Acupuncture

Acupuncture is a procedure in which a practitioner inserts needles into designated points on the skin. Some scientists believe that acupuncture triggers the release of the body's natural painkillers. Acupuncture has been shown to offer relief from chronic pain. Acupuncture is sometimes used by people with neuropathy, the painful nerve damage of diabetes.

Biofeedback

Biofeedback is a technique that helps a person become more aware of and learn to deal with the body's response to pain. This alternative therapy emphasizes relaxation and stress-reduction techniques. Some professionals who use biofeedback use guided imagery as a relaxation technique. With guided imagery, a person thinks of peaceful mental images, such as ocean waves. A person may also include the images of controlling or curing a chronic disease, such as diabetes. People using this technique believe their condition can be eased with these positive images.

Chromium

The benefit of added chromium for diabetes has been studied and debated for several years. Several studies report that chromium supplementation may improve diabetes control. Chromium is needed to make glucose tolerance factor, which helps improve the action of insulin. Because of insufficient information on the use of chromium to treat diabetes, no recommendations for supplementation yet exist.

Ginseng

Several types of plants are referred to as ginseng, but most studies of ginseng and diabetes have used American ginseng. Those studies have shown some glucose-lowering effects in fasting and post-prandial (after meal) blood glucose levels as well as in A1C levels (average blood glucose levels over a 3-month period). However, larger and more long-term studies are needed before general recommendations for use of ginseng can be made. Researchers also have determined that the amount of glucose-lowering compound in ginseng plants varies widely.

Magnesium

Although the relationship between magnesium and diabetes has been studied for decades, it is not yet fully understood. Studies suggest that a deficiency in magnesium may worsen blood glucose control in type 2 diabetes. Scientists believe that a deficiency of magnesium interrupts insulin secretion in the pancreas and increases insulin resistance in the body's tissues. Evidence suggests that a deficiency of magnesium may contribute to certain diabetes complications. A recent analysis showed that people with higher dietary intakes of magnesium (through consumption of whole grains, nuts, and green leafy vegetables) had a decreased risk of type 2 diabetes. With all of this being said, while increasing intake of magnesium may help those prone to and with diabetes, the true relationship is still not fully understood.

Vanadium

Vanadium is an element found in tiny amounts in plants and animals. Early studies showed that vanadium normalized blood glucose levels in animals with type 1 and type 2 diabetes. A recent study found that when people with diabetes were given vanadium, they developed a modest increase in insulin sensitivity and were able to decrease their insulin requirements. Currently researchers want to understand how vanadium works in the body, discover potential side effects, and establish safe dosages.

Be cautious when using herbal supplements. The potency, purity, and quality vary because supplements are not regulated by the Food and Drug Administration. Many also have a carbohydrate base to mix and stabilize the herbs can affect blood glucose levels in diabetics. Alternative and complimentary treatments should not replace conventional, proven treatments. Discuss with your doctor any plan to include supplements or alternative/complementary therapies in managing your diabetes. You should have this discussion before starting other treatments.

Lifestyle Changes

Of course, diabetes control takes more than a pill or a shot. It also takes effort on your part to adjust your lifestyle. All people with diabetes should follow a healthy food and physical activity plan (see Chapter 6). For type 1 diabetics, insulin is always needed, along with a well-defined treatment plan. In some type 2 diabetics, following a healthy food and exercise plan initially achieves diabetes control, but most will eventually require the addition of oral medications and/or insulin.

The exact methods of treatment—diet, exercise, oral antidiabetic agents and/or insulin—should be tailored to individual needs. People with diabetes should participate in the decision-making process, clearly stating options, goals, and targets.

5

Complications

Although it may seem to give a negative tone to what is intended to be a positive book, this discussion of the complications of uncontrolled diabetes should give you a healthy respect for the disease. Diabetics have a greater risk for the development of complications of various body systems due to the accumulation of glucose in the nerves and tissues of the body.

Blindness and Other Vision Problems

Blindness is 29 times more frequent in diabetics than in the general population. Diabetic retinopathy is the leading cause of blindness in adults in North America. The retina and nerves of the body do not require insulin to use glucose, and thus are susceptible to the damaging effects of high blood glucose concentrations. The accumulation of glucose in the retina and nerves leads to tissue and nerve dysfunction. Small hemorrhages are frequently seen after 5 years of type 1 diabetes. This can lead to large hemorrhages, scar formation, and eventual loss of vision. High blood glucose and high blood pressure from diabetes can hurt these four parts of your eye:

Retina (REH-ti-nuh). The retina is the lining at the back of the eye. The retina's job is to sense light coming into the eye.

Vitreous (VIH-tree-us). The vitreous is a jelly-like fluid that fills the back of the eye.

Lens. The lens is at the front of the eye and it focuses light on the retina.

Optic nerve. The optic nerve is the eye's main nerve to the brain.

The most common diabetes eye problem, diabetic retinopathy, results from damage to the retina. Diabetic damage to the retina happens slowly. The retinas have tiny blood vessels that are easy to damage. Having high blood glucose and high blood pressure for a long time can damage these tiny blood vessels. First, these tiny blood vessels swell and weaken. Some blood vessels then become clogged and do not let enough blood through. At first, you might not have any loss of sight from these changes, which is why you need to have a dilated eye exam once a year even if your sight seems fine.

As diabetes retina problems get worse, new blood vessels grow. These new blood vessels are weak. They break easily and leak blood into the vitreous of your eye. The leaking blood keeps light from reaching the retina. You may see floating spots or almost total darkness. Sometimes the blood will clear out by itself, but you might need surgery to remove it. Over the years, the swollen and weak blood vessels can form scar tissue and pull the retina away from the back of the eye. If the retina becomes detached, you may see floating spots or flashing lights. You may feel as if a curtain has been pulled over part of what you are looking at. A detached retina can cause loss of sight or blindness if you don't take care of it right away. Diabetes can result in two other eye problems—cataracts and glaucoma. People without diabetes can get these eye problems, too. But people with diabetes get them more often and at a younger age.

- A cataract (KA-ter-act) is a cloud over the lens of your eye, which is usually clear. The lens focuses light onto the retina. A cataract makes everything you look at seem cloudy. You need surgery to remove the cataract. During surgery, your lens is taken out and a plastic lens, like a contact lens, is put in. The plastic lens stays in your eye all the time. Cataract surgery helps you see clearly again.

- Glaucoma (glaw-KOH-muh) starts from pressure building up in the eye. Over time, this pressure damages your eye's main nerve—the optic nerve. The damage first causes you to lose sight from the sides of your eyes. Treating glaucoma is usually simple. Your eye doctor will give you special drops to use every day to lower the pressure in your eye. Or your eye doctor may want you to have laser surgery.

There are several steps you can take to prevent diabetes eye problems:

- Keep your blood glucose and blood pressure as close to normal as you can.

- Have an eye doctor examine your eyes once a year. Have this exam even if your vision is OK. The eye doctor will use drops to make the black part of your eyes (pupils) bigger. This is called dilating your pupil, which allows the doctor to see the back of your eye. Finding eye problems early and getting treatment right away will help prevent more serious problems later on.

- Ask your eye doctor to check for signs of cataracts and glaucoma.

- If you are pregnant and have diabetes, see an eye doctor during

your first 3 months.
- If you are planning to get pregnant, ask your doctor if you should have an eye exam.
- Don't smoke.

Kidney Disease

Renal (kidney) disease is 17 times more likely to occur in diabetics. Diabetic nephropathy, which occurs in one-third of type 1 diabetics, is a condition that leads to decreased filtration by the kidneys, loss of protein in the urine, and high blood pressure, and is the leading cause of end-stage renal disease.

Diabetic kidney disease takes many years to develop. In some people, the filtering function of the kidneys is actually higher than normal in the first few years of their diabetes. This process has been called hyperfiltration.

Over several years, people who are developing kidney disease will have small amounts of the blood protein albumin begin to leak into their urine. At its first stage, this condition has been called microalbuminuria. The kidney's filtration function usually remains normal during this period.

As the disease progresses, more albumin leaks into the urine. Various names are attached to this interval of the disease, such as overt diabetic nephropathy or macroalbuminuria. As the amount of albumin in the urine increases, filtering function usually begins to drop. The body retains various wastes as filtration falls. Creatinine is one such waste, and a blood test for creatinine can measure the decline in kidney filtration. As kidney damage develops, blood pressure often rises as well.

High blood pressure, or hypertension, is also a major factor in the development of kidney problems in people with diabetes. Both a family history of hypertension and the presence of hypertension appear to increase chances of developing kidney disease. Hypertension also accelerates the progress of kidney disease where it already exists. The American Diabetes Association and the National Heart, Lung, and Blood Institute recommend that people with diabetes keep their blood pressure below 130/80.

Overall, kidney damage rarely occurs in the first 10 years of diabetes, and usually 15 to 25 years will pass before kidney failure occurs. For people who live with diabetes for more than 25 years without any signs of kidney failure, the risk of ever developing it decreases.

Scientists have made great progress in developing methods that slow the onset and progression of kidney disease in people with diabetes. Drugs used to lower blood pressure (antihypertensive drugs) can slow the progression of kidney disease significantly. Two types of drugs (angiotensin-converting enzyme ACE inhibitors and angiotensin receptor blockers ARBs), have proven effective in slowing the progression of kidney disease. In addition, a diuretic is very useful. Beta blockers, calcium channel blockers, and other blood pressure drugs may also be needed.

In people with diabetes, excessive consumption of protein may be harmful. Experts recommend that people with kidney disease of diabetes consume the recommended dietary allowance (RDA) for protein, but avoid high-protein diets. For people with greatly reduced kidney function, a diet containing reduced amounts of protein may help delay the onset of kidney failure. Anyone following a reduced-protein diet should work with a dietitian to ensure adequate nutrition.

A third treatment, known as intensive management of blood glucose or glycemic control, has shown great promise for people with type 1 and type 2 diabetes, especially for those in early stages of nephropathy. The regimen includes testing blood glucose frequently, administering insulin frequently throughout the day on the basis of food intake and exercise, following a diet and exercise plan, and consulting a health care team frequently. Some people use an insulin pump to supply insulin throughout the day.

When people with diabetes experience kidney failure, they must undergo either dialysis or a kidney transplant. As recently as the 1970s, medical experts commonly excluded people with diabetes from dialysis and transplantation, in part because the experts felt damage caused by diabetes would offset benefits of the treatments. Today, because of better control of diabetes and improved rates of survival following treatment, doctors do not hesitate to offer dialysis and kidney transplantation to people with diabetes.

Neuropathy

If you have had diabetes for more than 15 years, than you need to be concerned with the possibility of developing neuropathy. Diabetic neuropathies are a family of nerve disorders caused by diabetes. Diabetes can, over time, damage nerves throughout the body. Neuropathies lead to numbness and sometimes pain and weakness in the hands, arms, feet, and legs. Problems may also occur in every organ system, including the digestive tract, heart, and sex organs. People with diabetes can develop nerve problems at any time, but the longer a person has diabetes, the greater the risk.

An estimated 50 percent of those with diabetes have some form of neuropathy, but not all with neuropathy have symptoms. The highest rates of neuropathy occur among people who have had the disease for at least 25 years.

Diabetic neuropathy also appears to be more common in people who have had problems controlling their blood glucose levels, in those with high levels of blood fat and blood pressure, in overweight people, and in people over the age of 40.

There are four different types of neuropathy: peripheral, autonomic, proximal, and focal.

Peripheral Neuropathy

Peripheral neuropathy damages nerves in the arms and legs. The feet and legs are likely to be affected before the hands and arms. Many people with diabetes have signs of neuropathy upon examination but have no symptoms at all. Symptoms of peripheral neuropathy may include:

- numbness or insensitivity to pain or temperature
- a tingling, burning, or prickling sensation
- sharp pains or cramps
- extreme sensitivity to touch, even a light touch
- loss of balance and coordination

These symptoms are often worse at night.

Peripheral neuropathy may also cause muscle weakness and loss of reflexes, especially at the ankle, leading to changes in gait (walking). Foot deformities, such as hammertoes and the collapse of the midfoot, may occur. Blisters and sores may appear on numb areas of the foot because pressure or injury goes unnoticed. If foot injuries are not treated promptly, the infection may spread to the bone, and the foot may then have to be amputated. Some experts estimate that half of all such amputations are preventable if minor problems are caught and treated in time.

Problems with blood circulation in the legs, called peripheral vascular disease, may also be a problem and can cause leg pain. Exercise may increase the pain—however exercise helps improve blood circulation, so the very thing that causes pain is actually good for you. You'll need to exercise for shorter periods of time, just until you feel pain, and then rest for a minute or two. Once the pain stops, continue with the exercise. Take rests as you need during exercise. This is called interval training and is perfect for diabetics with peripheral vascular disease.

Autonomic Neuropathy

Autonomic neuropathy affects the nerves that control the heart, regulate blood pressure, and control blood glucose levels. It also affects other internal organs, causing problems with digestion, respiratory function, urination, sexual response, and vision. In addition, the system that restores blood glucose levels to normal after a hypoglycemic episode may be affected, resulting in loss of the warning signs of hypoglycemia such as sweating and palpitations.

Unawareness of Hypoglycemia. Normally, symptoms such as shakiness occur as blood glucose levels drop below 70 mg/dL. In people with autonomic neuropathy, symptoms may not occur, making hypoglycemia difficult to recognize. However, other problems can also cause hypoglycemia unawareness so this does not always indicate nerve damage.

Heart and Circulatory System. The heart and circulatory system are part of the cardiovascular system, which controls blood circulation. Damage to nerves in the cardiovascular system interferes with the body's ability to adjust blood pressure and heart rate. As a result, blood pressure may drop sharply after sitting or standing, causing a person to feel light-headed—or even to faint. It is important when changing from floor exercises to standing exercises to rise slowly. Sit upright for a few seconds. Come up to a kneeling position, pausing for another few seconds, and gradually rise to a standing position. This may help prevent dizziness. Damage to the nerves that control your heart rate can mean that it remains high, instead of rising and falling in response to your normal body functions and exercise.

Digestive System. Nerve damage to the digestive system most commonly causes constipation. Damage can also cause the stomach to empty too slowly, a condition called gastroparesis. Severe gastroparesis can lead to persistent nausea and vomiting, bloating, and loss of appetite. Gastroparesis can make blood glucose levels fluctuate widely as well, due to abnormal food digestion. Nerve damage to the esophagus may make swallowing difficult, while nerve damage to the bowels can cause constipation alternating with frequent, uncontrolled diarrhea, especially at night. Problems with the digestive system may lead to weight loss.

Urinary Tract and Sex Organs. Autonomic neuropathy most often affects the organs that control urination and sexual function. Nerve damage can prevent the bladder from emptying completely, allowing bacteria to grow in the bladder and kidneys and causing urinary tract infections. When the nerves of the bladder are damaged, urinary incontinence may result because a person may not be able to sense when the bladder is full or control the muscles that release urine. Neuropathy can also gradually decrease sexual response in men and women, although the sex drive is unchanged. A man may be unable to have erections or may reach sexual climax without ejaculating normally. A woman may have difficulty with lubrication, arousal, or orgasm.

Sweat Glands. Autonomic neuropathy can affect the nerves that control sweating. When nerve damage prevents the sweat glands from working properly, the body cannot regulate its temperature properly. Nerve damage can also cause profuse sweating at night or while eating.

Eyes. Finally, autonomic neuropathy can affect the pupils of the eyes, making them less responsive to changes in light. As a result, a person may not be able to see well when the light is turned on in a dark room or may have trouble driving at night

Proximal Neuropathy

Proximal neuropathy, sometimes called lumbosacral plexus neuropathy, femoral neuropathy, or diabetic amyotrophy, starts with pain in either the thighs, hips, buttocks, or legs, usually on one side of the body. This type of neuropathy is more common in those with type 2 diabetes and in older people. It causes weakness in the legs, manifested by an inability to go from a sitting to a standing position without help. Treatment for weakness or pain is usually needed. The length of the recovery period varies, depending on the type of nerve damage.

Focal Neuropathy

Occasionally, neuropathy appears suddenly and affects specific nerves, most often in the head, torso, or leg.

Focal neuropathy may cause:
- inability to focus the eye
- double vision
- aching behind one eye
- paralysis on one side of the face (Bell's palsy)
- severe pain in the lower back or pelvis
- pain in the front of a thigh
- pain in the chest, stomach, or flank
- pain on the outside of the shin or inside the foot
- chest or abdominal pain that is sometimes mistaken for heart disease, heart attack, or appendicitis

Focal neuropathy is painful and unpredictable and occurs most often in older people. However, it tends to improve by itself over weeks or months and does not cause long-term damage.

People with diabetes also tend to develop nerve compressions, also called entrapment syndromes. One of the most common is carpal tunnel syndrome, which causes numbness and tingling of the hand and sometimes muscle weakness or pain. Other nerves susceptible to entrapment may cause pain on the outside of the shin or the inside of the foot.

Cardiovascular Disease

Diabetics have a greater risk of developing cardiovascular disease than non-diabetics. This risk is greater in females than in males. High blood pressure can damage the heart and blood vessels. Heart and blood vessel disease can lead to heart attacks and strokes, which are the leading causes of death for people with diabetes. The lining of the blood vessels, which is usually smooth, tends to get rough in diabetics, perhaps in response to high concentrations of glucose circulating in the blood. A rough surface causes platelets to stick to the walls of the arteries. Eventually a build up of platelets causes the arteries to narrowing restricting blood flow through the vessels and reduce blood flow to the hands and feet. When tissues do not get enough blood flow tissue death occurs. It is for this reason that diabetics are 5 times more likely to have a leg or toe amputated.

6

Diet and Weight Control

This chapter will help you learn more about eating healthy. It starts with the Food Guide Pyramid. After you have an understanding of what and how much you should be eating, talk to your doctor or a dietitian about formulating a meal plan that's right for you.

The major nutritional goal for managing your diabetes is maintaining an appropriate weight. For most diabetics, this means weight loss. Keeping cholesterol levels within normal range and eating a healthy, nutritious diet are also very important. Your diet should be tailored to your individual needs and goals. However, general nutrition guidelines for diabetics are as follows:

Protein: 10 to 20 percent of total calories consumed should consist of proteins from animal and/or vegetable sources. (If you have nephropathy, a protein intake of 0.8 g/kg or 10 percent of total calories is recommended.)

Fats: Intake is dependent upon your medical history and treatment goals. Fat should provide less than 10 percent of total calories if you are obese, have high cholesterol, or are at risk for cardiovascular disease.

If you have normal cholesterol levels, 30 percent of total calories should come from polyunsaturated fats. Cholesterol intake should be limited to 300 mg or less.

Carbohydrates: 60 percent of calories should come from mostly complex carbohydrates.

Type 1 Diabetes

Type 1 diabetics should be as consistent as possible with regard to the time and frequency of meals and snacks. The amount of calories and carbohydrates consumed should be timed with peak insulin action. Since exercise lowers blood glucose levels, the time to exercise should be within two hours after eating your meal. After that, you risk the chance of going hypoglycemic.

You may need to consume 10 to 15 g of extra carbohydrates (piece of fruit or starch) for each hour of moderate exercise (for example, playing a round of golf) or 20 to 30 g of extra carbohydrates for each hour of vigorous exercise (for example, playing basketball).

Type 2 Diabetes

Since most type 2 diabetics are overweight, a modest calorie-restricted, low-fat diet, which will allow approximately one pound per week of weight loss, is appropriate. Space your meals four to five hours apart to avoid fluctuations in glucose levels. You may want to consult with a nutritionist to develop a meal plan that is tailored to your condition.

Keeping Your Blood Glucose at a Healthy Level

Whether you have type 1 or type 2 diabetes, what, when, and how much you eat all affect your blood glucose. Blood glucose is the main sugar found in the blood and the body's main source of energy. If you have diabetes (or impaired glucose tolerance), your blood glucose can go too high if you eat too much. If your blood glucose goes too high, you can get sick. Your blood glucose can also go too high or drop too low if you don't take the right amount of diabetes medications. If your blood glucose stays high too much of the time, you can get heart, eye, foot, kidney, and other problems. You can also have problems if your blood glucose gets too low (hypoglycemia).

Keeping your blood glucose at a healthy level will prevent or postpone diabetes problems. Ask your doctor or diabetes teacher what a healthy blood glucose level is for you. For most people, target blood glucose levels are 90 to 130 before meals and less than 180 1 to 2 hours after the start of a meal.

These steps can help you keep your blood glucose at a healthy level.

- Eat about the same amount of food each day.
- Eat your meals and snacks at about the same times each day.
- It is important to eat the same amount of food at the same time every day because your blood glucose goes up after you eat. If you eat a big lunch one day and a small lunch the next day, your blood glucose levels will fluctuate too much.
- Keep your blood glucose at a healthy level by eating about the same amount of carbohydrate foods at about the same times each day. Carbohydrate foods, also called carbs, provide glucose for energy. Starches, fruits, milk, starchy vegetables such as corn, and sweets are all carbohydrate foods.
- Talk with your doctor or diabetes teacher about how many meals

and snacks to eat each day.

- Do not skip meals or snacks.
- Take your medicines at the same times each day.
- What you eat and when affects how your diabetes medicines work. Talk with your doctor or diabetes teacher about the best times to take your diabetes medicines based on your meal plan.
- Exercise at about the same times each day.
- What you eat and when also depend on how much you exercise. Exercise is an important part of staying healthy and controlling your blood glucose. Physical activity should be safe and enjoyable, so be sure to talk with your doctor about what types of exercise are right for you.

You can also help control your blood glucose and diabetes by staying at a healthy weight, a result of eating healthy and getting enough exercise. A healthy weight also helps you control your cholesterol and lower your blood pressure.

Most of the time you will want to avoid rapid elevations in blood glucose levels. But there are times—for example, if you become hypoglycemic—when you may want your levels to rise more quickly. It is important to pay attention to the glycemic index of the food you eat. Glycemic index refers to the rate at which blood glucose levels are affected.

The Diabetes Food Pyramid

Using the Diabetes Food Pyramid helps you eat a variety of healthy foods. Variety means eating foods from each of the food groups every day. When you eat different foods each day, you get the vitamins and minerals you need. The pyramid is divided into six groups. You should eat more foods from the largest group at the base of the pyramid and less from the smaller groups at the top of the pyramid. The number of servings needed every day is not the same for everyone, so a range of servings is given to ensure you get the foods you need for good health.

What is the right number of servings for you?

The Diabetes Food Pyramid gives a range of servings for each group, but it is only a guide. If you have diabetes, a dietitian can design a specific meal plan for you.

The following table gies you examples of low, moderate, and high glycemic index foods.

Low Glycemic Index	Moderate Glycemic Index	High Glycemic Index
fiber/bran cereal	whole-wheat bread	bagels, pita bread
unsweetened low-fat yogurt	oatmeal	white bread
apples	corn	Cherrios
cherries	sweet potatoes	shredded wheat cereal
peaches	brown rice	frozen yogurt
pears	low-fat fruit yogurt	white rice
plums	apple juice	carrots
red beans	grapes	bananas
lentils	oranges	mangos
spaghetti	dried apricots	orange juice
tomatoes	chickpeas (canned)	raisins
spinach	sweet corn	
asparagus	french fries	
broccoli	peas (canned)	
penuts	chips	
almonds	crackers	
walnuts		

Remember that the number of servings listed is for the entire day. Since food raises blood sugar levels, it is best to space servings throughout the day. For example, 4 servings of fruit might be divided between 3 meals and 1 snack.

Grains, Beans, and Starchy Vegetables: **6 or more servings/day**
(good source of B vitamins and fiber)

Fruits: **3–4 servings/day**
(contain vitamins C, A, potassium, folate, and fiber)

Vegetables: **3–5 servings/day**
(provide vitamins A, C, folate, and fiber)

Milk: **2–3 servings/day**
(source of calcium, protein, vitamins A and D)

Meats: **2–3 servings/day**
(good source of iron, zinc, B vitamins, and protein)

Fats, Sweets, and Alcohol:
The foods at the tip of the pyramid should be eaten in small amounts. Fats and oils should be limited because they are high in calories. Sweets are high in sugar and should be eaten only once in a while.

What is a serving size in the Food Pyramid?

Each of the following represents one serving from each of the food groups in the Diabetes Food Pyramid:

Grains, Beans, and Starchy Vegetables:
1 slice of bread; 1/2 small bagel, English muffin, or bun; 1/2 cup cooked cereal, pasta, rice; 3/4 cup ready-to-eat cereal; 1/2 cup cooked dried beans, corn, peas

Vegetable Group:
1 cup raw vegetable; 1/2 cup vegetable juice

Fruit Group:
1 medium-size fresh fruit; 1/2 cup canned fruit; 1/2 cup fruit juice

Milk Group:
1 cup (8 ounces) milk or yogurt

Meat Group:

2–3 ounces cooked lean meat, skinless poultry, or fish; 1 egg; 2 tablespoons peanut butter; 2–3 ounces cheese

Fats, Sweets, and Alcohol:

1 teaspoon butter, margarine, or mayonnaise; 1 tablespoon cream cheese or salad dressing; 1/2 cup ice cream.

What to do when eating combined foods

Many dishes are made up of several types of foods. Therefore, they do not fit in one specific group. The meal planner will help you to measure using foods from the Diabetes Food Pyramid.

	GRAINS/BEANS/ STARCHY VEGETABLE	VEGETABLE	MEAT	FAT
Spanish Omelet	1		1	1/2
Beef or Turkey Stew	1		1	1
Caribbean Red Snapper			1	1 1/2
Two-Cheese Pizza	2		1	1 1/2
Eggplant Lasagna	1		1	1
Rice with Chicken, Spanish Style	1 1/2	1	1	1
Seafood Stew			2	1/2

This is just an example. If you have diabetes, consult a registered dietitian to help you make your own meal plan. Your meal plan will be based on many factors, including your weight goal, height, age, and physical activity. The following Sample Meal Plan includes 3 meals and 2 snacks, with suggested servings.

Grains, Beans, and Starchy Vegetables

This category contains bread, grains, cereal, pasta, and starchy vegetables like corn and potatoes. They give your body energy, vitamins, minerals, and fiber. Whole grain starches are healthier because they have more vitamins, minerals, and fiber.

Eat some starches at each meal. People might tell you not to eat starches, but that is not correct. Eating starches is healthy for everyone, including people with diabetes. Examples of starches include bread, pasta, corn, potatoes, rice, crackers, tortillas, beans, and yams.

If you have more than one serving at a meal, you can choose several different starches or have two or three servings of one starch. Here are some healthy ways to eat starches:

- Buy whole grain breads and cereals.
- Eat fewer fried and high-fat starches such as regular tortilla chips and potato chips, french fries, pastries, or biscuits. Try pretzels, fat-free popcorn, baked tortilla or potato chips, baked potatoes, or low-fat muffins.
- Use low-fat yogurt, fat-free yogurt, or fat-free sour cream instead of regular sour cream on a baked potato.
- Use mustard instead of mayonnaise on a sandwich.
- Use low-fat or fat-free substitutes such as low-fat mayonnaise or light margarine on bread, rolls, or toast.
- Eat cereal with fat-free (skim) or low-fat (1%) milk.

SAMPLE MEAL PLAN FOR A DAY

MEAL	FOOD PYRAMID GROUP SERVINGS	SUGGESTED MENU
BREAKFAST	Fruit (1)	Fresh orange
	Grains/Beans/Starchy Veg. (2)	1 medium baked plantain
	Milk (1)	1 cup 1% low-fat Milk
	Fat (1)	Oil, 1 teaspoon
LUNCH	Meat (1)	Two-cheese pizza
	Grains/Beans/Starchy Veg. (2)	2 slices (see recipe)
	Fat (1)	
	Fruit (1)	Melon, 1 cup/cubed
	Vegetable (1)	Mixed green salad
AFTERNOON SNACK	Fruit (1)	Apple, 1 medium
	Meat (1)	Peanut butter, 2 tablespoons
	Grains/Beans/Starchy Veg. (1)	Whole wheat crackers, 5
DINNER	Grains/Beans/Starchy Veg. (1)	Rice with Chicken Spanish Style
	Meat (1)	1 cup (see recipe)
	Vegetable (1)	
	Fat (1)	
	Fruit (1)	Pineapple rings, 1/2 cup
	Vegetable (1)	Spinach, 1 cup raw
	Fat (1)	Vinaigrette, 1 tablespoon
EVENING SNACK	Milk (1)	Yogurt, low-fat, 1 cup
	Grains/Beans/Starchy Veg. (1)	Bread sticks, 2

Vegetable Group

Vegetables are healthy for everyone, including people with diabetes. Eat raw and cooked vegetables every day. Vegetables give you vitamins, minerals, and fiber with very few calories. Look for vegetables that are bright in color. A few examples are: carrots, peppers, eggplants, broccoli, tomatoes, and spinach.

Here are some healthy ways to eat vegetables:

- Eat raw and cooked vegetables with little or no fat, sauces, or dressings.
- Try low-fat or fat-free salad dressing on raw vegetables or salads.
- Steam vegetables using a small amount of water or low-fat broth.
- Mix in some chopped onion or garlic.
- Use a little vinegar or some lemon or lime juice.
- Add a small piece of lean ham or smoked turkey instead of fat to vegetables when cooking.
- Sprinkle with herbs and spices. These flavorings add almost no fat or calories.
- If you do use a small amount of fat, use canola oil, olive oil, or soft margarines (liquid or tub types) instead of fat from meat, butter, or shortening.

Fruit Group

Fruit, like vegetables, is healthy for everyone, including people with diabetes. Fruit gives you energy, vitamins and minerals, and fiber.

Here are some healthy suggestions for eating fruit:

- Eat fruits raw or cooked, as juice with no sugar added, canned in their own juice, or dried.
- Buy smaller pieces of fruit.
- Eat pieces of fruit rather than drinking fruit juice. Pieces of fruit are more filling.

• Drink fruit juice in small amounts.
• Save high-sugar and high-fat fruit desserts such as peach cobbler or cherry pie for special occasions.

Milk Group

Fat-free and low-fat milk and yogurt are healthy for everyone, including people with diabetes. Milk and yogurt give you energy, protein, calcium, vitamin A, and other vitamins and minerals. Drink fat-free (skim or nonfat) or low-fat (1%) milk each day. Eat low-fat or fat-free yogurt.

Here are some healthy ways to eat your milk and yogurt:
• Eat low-fat or fat-free fruit yogurt sweetened with a low-calorie sweetener.
• Use low-fat plain yogurt as a substitute for sour cream.

Meat Group

This food group contains meat (beef, pork, lamb), chicken, turkey, eggs, fish, nuts, and tofu or soy products. Eat small amounts of some of these foods each day. All these foods provide our bodies with protein. Protein foods help your body build tissue and muscles. They also give your body vitamins and minerals.

Here are some healthy ways to eat food from this group:
• Buy cuts of beef, pork, ham, and lamb that have only a little fat on them. Trim off extra fat.
• Eat chicken or turkey without the skin.
• Cook meat or meat substitutes in low-fat ways (broil, grill, stir-fry, roast, steam, or stew).
• To add more flavor, use vinegars, lemon juice, soy or teriyaki sauce, salsa, ketchup, barbecue sauce, and herbs and spices.

- Cook eggs with a small amount of fat or use cooking spray.
- Limit the amounts of nuts, peanut butter, and fried chicken that you eat. They are high in fat.
- Choose low-fat or fat-free cheese.

Fats, Sweets, and Alcohol

This group includes butter, margarine, lard, and oils that we add to foods and use to cook foods. Some oils are canola, olive, and vegetable. Fats are also found in meats, dairy products, snack foods, and some sweets. To control your diabetes, it is best to eat foods with less fat, especially saturated fat.

Sweets are sugary foods that have calories but not very many vitamins and minerals. Some sweets are also high in fat—like cakes, pies, and cookies. Eating too many sugary and high-fat foods makes it hard to control your blood sugar and weight. If you do eat fats and sweets, eat small portions.

Alcohol has calories but no nutrients. If you drink alcohol on an empty stomach, it can make your blood glucose level too low. It can also raise your blood fats.

It's okay to have sweets or alcohol once in a while. Try having sugar-free popsicles, diet soda, fat-free ice cream or frozen yogurt, or sugar-free hot cocoa mix.

Other tips:
- Share desserts in restaurants.
- Order small or child-size servings of ice cream or frozen yogurt.
- Divide homemade desserts into small servings and wrap each individually. Freeze extra servings.
- Don't keep dishes of candy in the house or at work.
- Don't drink alcohol on an empty stomach.

Caloric Guidelines

The amount of food you should eat day varies from person to person, depending on various factors. Here are some guidelines.

Have about 1,200 to 1,600 calories a day if you are:
- a small woman who exercises
- a small or medium woman who wants to lose weight
- a medium woman who does not exercise much

Choose this many servings from these food groups to have 1,200 to 1,600 calories a day:

6 starches	2 milk and yogurt
3 vegetables	2 meat or meat substitute
2 fruit	up to 3 fats

Have about 1,600 to 2,000 calories a day if you are:
- a large woman who wants to lose weight
- a small man at a healthy weight
- a medium man who does not exercise much
- a medium to large man who wants to lose weight

Choose this many servings from these food groups to have 1,600 to 2,000 calories a day:

8 starches	2 milk and yogurt
4 vegetables	2 meat or meat substitute
3 fruit	up to 4 fats

Have about 2,000 to 2,400 calories a day if you are:
- a medium to large man who does a lot of exercise or has a physically active job
- a large man at a healthy weight
- a large woman who exercises a lot or has a physically active job

Choose this many servings from these food groups to have 2,000 to 2,400 calories a day:

11 starches	2 milk and yogurt
4 vegetables	2 meat or meat substitute
3 fruit	up to 5 fats

Measuring Your Food

Sometimes it's hard to measure food. When you're at home it's a bit easier. You can use these tools to make sure your food servings are the right size:
- measuring cups
- measuring spoons
- a food scale

Also, the nutrition facts label on food packages tells you how much of that food is in one serving.

Here are some other tips that will help you choose the right serving sizes:
- Measure a serving size of dry cereal or hot cereal, pasta, or rice and pour it into a bowl or plate. The next time you eat that food, use the same bowl or plate and fill it to the same level.
- For one serving of milk, measure 1 cup and pour it into a glass. See how high it fills the glass. Always drink milk out of that size glass.
- Meat weighs more before it's cooked. For example, 4 ounces of

raw meat will weigh about 3 ounces after cooking. For meat with a bone, like a pork chop or chicken leg, cook 5 ounces raw to get 3 ounces cooked.

When you aren't able to measure your food, these hints can help you estimate the amount you are eating.

- One serving of meat or meat substitute is about the size and thickness of the palm of your hand or a deck of cards.
- A small fist is equal to about 1/2 cup of fruit, vegetables, or starches like rice.
- A small fist is equal to 1 small piece of fresh fruit.
- A thumb is equal to about 1 ounce of meat or cheese.
- The tip of a thumb is equal to about 1 teaspoon.

7

Benefits of Exercise for Diabetics

It is a well-known fact that exercise has many health benefits, particularly for the prevention of coronary artery disease. These benefits can also help to prevent and treat type 2 diabetes if you are at high risk or have a family history of the disease. As we have learned, diabetics are frequently obese and inactive, and have high blood pressure and high cholesterol. If you can improve those risk factors through exercise, and make positive changes in body fat, activity levels, blood pressure, and diet, you should see an improvement in your diabetes. Exercise improves the uptake of glucose both during and after exercise. Surprisingly, long after you stop exercising, glucose uptake is elevated. The affect of exercise on insulin sensitivity can last up to 16 hours before it begins to slowly decline.

Some of the benefits of exercise for Type 2 diabetics are listed below:

- Reduced blood glucose levels
- Improved glucose tolerance
- Improved insulin from glucose taken by mouth
- Improved cholesterol levels
- Decreased blood pressure
- Deceased risk of cardiovascular disease
- Improved overall fitness and energy levels
- Increased calorie burning which will decrease body weight
- Improved well-being and self-esteem
- Improved strength and flexibility.

Blood Sugar Levels and Exercise

The American College of Sports Medicine (ACSM) offers the following guidelines for monitoring blood glucose levels. Your should monitor your blood glucose levels before, during, and after exercise (every 15 minutes postexercise). If your blood sugar measures above 250mg/dl, and ketones are present in your urine or if it is greater than 300mg/dl, postpone your exercise session until your glucose levels come down. If your blood glucose is lower than normal, or less than 100mg/dl, you should eat a piece of fruit or a readily absorbed carbohydrate before exercise and have carbohydrates, such as fruit juice, available during and after exercise.

Regarding your insulin requirements with exercise, ACSM suggests you decrease intermediate-acting insulin by 30 to 35 percent on the day of exercise. With intermediate and short-acting insulin you should omit your dose of short-acting insulin before exercise. In the case of multiple doses of short-acting insulin, you should reduce the dose by 30 to 35 percent, and eat a carbohydrate before exercise. You should also not exercise at the time of peak insulin action. These are, however, general guidelines and you should check with your doctor for specific recommendations as they relate to you.

It is important to keep a daily log of your glucose readings and the times you tested yourself. Include in your record book the times of your meals and the times and duration of your exercise sessions. With this information you can get an idea of the pattern of your blood glucose levels and the possible causes for abnormal levels. Review this information with your doctor to plan the best course of action to correct any problems. You may need to adjust your meals or the timing or intensity of your exercises accordingly.

Part II: Exercises for Diabetes

8

Exercise Recommendations for Diabetics

At this point, I hope you are convinced that exercise is the magic potion that will transform your life. With the exercise guidelines and exercise programs provided, you will be making a significant contribution to controlling your diabetes. In addition, you will increase your bone density and improve the function of your heart and muscles, not to mention boost your energy and self-esteem.

However, knowing the value of exercise doesn't mean you actually will exercise. Many people know they should exercise, but still remain sedentary. And the excuse most people give for not exercising is a lack of time. Did you know that if you accumulate at least 30 minutes of moderate intensity exercise most days of the week you can reap all the health benefits mentioned in this book? Moderate intensity can be described as fairly light to somewhat hard, or causing a heart rate of approximately 60 to 80 percent of your maximal heart rate.

What you can do is make exercise more compatible with your schedule. Exercise while you watch television; instead of driving the car to the corner store, walk. If you use a coin laundry, bring along your weights and strength train while you wash and dry your clothes. If you spend weekends at your kids' soccer games, walk the perimeter of the field as you watch the game instead of sitting on the sidelines. Do you get the idea? These suggestions can get your wheels in motion, and get you thinking of other ways you can incorporate exercise into your schedule. You have to make exercise a priority. Your health is worth it. The bottom line is, no matter what your approach, exercise has to become a habit. Just as you set the time aside to watch your favorite TV show, make exercise a part of your routine.

You need a daily dose of exercise the same way you need medicine. Exercise enhances your glucose metabolism and does a great job of lowering your circulating blood glucose. One bout of exercise can actually improve the glucose uptake by your cells for up to 16 hours. By making exercise a regular routine, over time, you can keep the levels consistently lower.

Before You Begin

Before beginning an exercise program, you must speak with your doctor about the appropriate screening and the necessity for an exercise stress test. Cardiac stress testing is recommended if you are 40 years old or over, if you have had type 2 diabetes for 10 years, or if you have had type 1 diabetes for 15 years.

It's recommended you follow these screening procedures before beginning an exercise program:
1. Review of medical history and complete physical

2. Diabetes evaluation: HbA1 (Glycosylated hemoglobin) test, eye exam, neurologic exam, urine test (check for protein in urine), nutritional evaluation
3. Cardiovascular Evaluation: blood pressure test, circulation evaluation (check pulses on lower leg) EKG, EKG exercise stress test, cholesterol testing.

If you have other medical conditions, those issues need to be addressed as well. The three primary goals of your exercise program are:
1. Reduce weight.
2. Eat a healthy diet that will promote weight loss (if needed) and good health. Fiber intake should be increased to 15 grams per 1,000 calories. Total fat intake should be less than 30 percent of your total calories intake, and saturated fat limited to less than 10 percent of your total calories.
3. Engage in continuous, moderate exercise, such as biking, swimming, or walking for 30 minutes per day.

A diabetic's exercise program should be kept at a predictable and consistent level of calorie expenditure to keep blood glucose levels regulated. High intensity, exhaustive, anaerobic, sprinting-type exercises should be avoided since these could result in a rapid drop in blood sugar. Exercising will cause you to use more blood sugar than remaining at rest. You must be careful to exercise at the appropriate intensity and monitor your blood sugar before, during, and after exercise to be certain it stays within the recommended ranges. You should also monitor your heart rate during exercise to make sure you are not exceeding your training heart rate range. You can monitor your heart rate by wearing a heart rate monitor or by taking your pulse. (See appendix TK) Diabetics are likely to reach their target heart rate quickly so it is important to give yourself an extended warmup (10 to 15 minutes) and gradually increase the workout's intensity. If you experience reduced sensation in your fingertips or have difficulty taking your pulse, you may use the perceived exertion scale to monitor the intensity of your exercise.

Foot Care

Before you begin, get yourself a good pair of sneakers from a reliable sporting goods store. Find a knowledgeable salesperson who can

Exercising Tips

1. Keep a sufficient source of sugar, fruit juice, or hard candy with you when you exercise in case of an insulin reaction.

2. Hypoglycemia (low blood sugar) can be a problem for several hours after a workout. Your muscles continue to use blood sugar after the exercise has ended in order to replenish glycogen stores. You should continue checking your blood sugar levels after exercise and know the signs of hypoglycemia. (Symptoms of hypoglycemia are sweating, hunger, palpitations, headache, fast heart rate, anxiety, tremor, dizziness, blurred vision, confusion, fainting, and coma. Exercise factors that contribute to hypoglycemia are: high-intensity exercise, longer exercise time, insufficient calorie intake prior to exercise, taking too much insulin, injecting insulin into a working muscle, and cold temperatures.)

3. Alcohol increases the chance of hypoglycemia. You should not exercise after drinking alcohol.

4. Do not exercise 60 to 90 minutes after an insulin injection or when insulin action has reached its peak.

5. As your fitness level improves, you may need to increase your calorie intake in order to provide energy for your increased energy needs.

6. Consider wearing a medical alert bracelet identifying you as a diabetic.

7. You may want to find an exercise partner who understands what to do if you should become hypoglycemic.

assist you in purchasing a supportive, properly fitting pair of shoes. Explain the type of exercise or activity that you will be performing since many sneakers are designed for specific purposes.

When you have diabetes, it is very important to take care of your feet. High blood sugar can damage the nerves in your feet and can cause blood flow problems. Caring for your feet means choosing a properly fitting, supportive sneaker. Would you ever use woolen mittens to take a hot dish from the oven? Probably not! Woolen

If you become hypoglycemic:

• Call 911.

• A fast-acting, high glycemic index carbohydrate should be consumed immediately.

• If available, measure your blood glucose with a glucose monitoring device.

• If your blood glucose is less than 70mg/dl, you will need 15gm of carbohydrate (3 to 4 glucose tablets, 1/2 cup of fruit juice, approximately 6 saltine crackers, or 1 tablespoon of sugar). Repeat testing every 15 minutes to check if glucose levels have returned to normal.

• You should not inject insulin into the major muscles that will be used during exercise. When you exercise an extremity muscle, such as the leg in running or cycling, the blood supply to that muscle increases, which consequently increases the rate of absorption of insulin. You want to have a steady rate of absorption; therefore the abdomen is the best injection site.

• Schedule exercise one to two hours after a meal, or when hypoglycemia medication is not at its peak activity.

• If you have insulin-dependent diabetes, you may need to adjust your insulin dose or diet on the days you exercise. General recommendation is to decrease insulin by 10 to 30 percent, depending on your glucose level, or eat a piece of fruit for each 30 minutes of aerobic exercise and one portion of protein for aerobic exercise lasting longer than one hour.

mittens were not designed for that purpose. So, why would you wear a casual sneaker for the purpose of exercising?

When you are actively engaged in exercise or sports, you place an increased demand on your feet. Your sneaker needs to provide good shock absorption and support. The fit of the sneaker should be correct so your foot is not constricted and is prevented from shifting around. Diabetics are prone to losing sensation in their feet. In that case you may not feel the pain and pressure associated with a poorly fitted sneaker. Ths can lead to the development of sores and blisters. The sore can easily become infected. Infection and poor blood flow can lead to amputation. As an operating room nurse, I have witnessed this sequence of events all too often. Signs of poor blood flow can include pain in your legs and feet, especially when you exercise, or legs that hurt during the night.

If you have ever visited a sporting goods store you have probably noticed the huge selection of sneakers to choose from. You should seek the help of a knowledgeable salesperson who can guide you to select the appropriate sneaker. You need to choose a sneaker that is designed for a specific activity. The best way to make a good choice is to understand the differences among the sneakers. A lot has to do with the purpose of the sneaker. The following list identifies characteristics of different sneakers:

Running. A running sneaker will have cushioning in the heel and mid-foot areas. The heel is elevated to protect the Achilles tendon. The mid-sole is designed to limit the medial rotation of the foot. The primary purpose of running sneaker design is motion control. The sole, however, has flexibility to allow the rolling motion of the foot to occur.

Walking. Walking produces less impact on the feet than running. In running, the vertical impact forces can be three times your body weight as opposed to 1.5 times your body weight with walking. The foot strike of walking differs from that of running; there is a more pronounced heel strike in walking. Walking sneakers are stiffer across the middle of the sole because flexibility is not as important in walking as it is in running. This feature provides greater stability.

Aerobics. High-impact aerobics can generate vertical impact forces similar to running. However, the impact forces are delivered mostly to the forefoot. Low-impact aerobics produces less of an impact force. Sneakers designed for aerobic dance tend to focus more on lateral support in addition to cushioning the foot. These sneakers tend to be firmer in the midsoles which provides stability, and also have reinforced heel counters.

Weight Training. For fitness or weight-training activities, a simple court shoe (tennis or racquetball sneaker) is usually adequate. Cushioning is not as important as stability. You should remember to use free weights on a carpeted floor. A firm, stable base of support is very important. Cushioning found in aerobic or running shoes may lead to instability injuries when used for weight training.

Cross Training. Shoe manufacturers are producing cross training, or multi-purpose, sneakers. Cross trainers will have more cushioning, especially in the heel, which allows them to be used for running. However, they don't typically have the same heel design as running sneakers. Because they have lateral support and thicker leather uppers they tend to be a little heavier and bulkier than most running sneakers. Most cross-trainers function well for aerobic exercises. They may be the best choice, especially if you are overweight.

Over time, any sneaker breaks down and loses support and cushioning features. Generally, you should replace your sneakers every four months. Keep in mind that lighter-weight shoes collapse more easily and cause injury more than heavier shoes.

Tips for Foot Care

1. You should inspect your feet daily. Check for cracks, blisters, and cuts.
2. Wash your feet daily with warm water and mild soap. Dry your feet well, especially between the toes.
3. You can use lotion on your feet but not between the toes.
4. File your toenails straight across with an emery board.
5. Shake out your shoes and socks before you put them on. You don't want to have small pebbles or anything pressing on your feet.
6. Wear shoes that fit well and are comfortable.
7. Don't go barefoot!
8. Choose cotton or wool socks to keep your feet dry.
9. Heating pads and hot water bottles can be harmful when used on the feet, especially if you have reduced sensation in your feet.
10. Never cut corns or calluses. See your doctor for the treatment of corns, calluses, or warts.

Types of Exercise

Diabetics who exercise are aiming for weight loss, which means an improvement in body composition, or a reduction in body fat and an increase in lean muscle mass. This could potentially regulate your glucose levels and decrease risk factors for heart disease. You can accomplish this through a combination of aerobic conditioning (any activity that is continuous, rhythmic in nature and uses the large muscles of the body over 20 to 60 minutes) and resistance training (using lower weights with 10 to 15 repetitions to strengthen your muscles). The exercises offered in this book can be divided into three categories: stretching, aerobic conditioning, and resistance training. Each has different purposes and effects on the body, but all are equally important.

Stretching

Stretching is always a good idea. Regularly stretching your muscles will improve your flexibility and range of motion. Stretching before and after physical activities may prevent injuries and muscle soreness. When you stretch before you exercise, hold the stretches for approximately 10 seconds to prepare the muscles and joints for the workout to follow. When you stretch at the end of exercise, hold the stretches for 20 to 30 seconds to improve flexibility and ultimately increase the resting length of the muscle. Improvements in flexibility occur with the stretches after exercise because it is really more beneficial to stretch a muscle when it is warmed up.

The recommendations for flexibility training are:

Frequency: 2 to 3 sessions per week

Hold each stretch to the point of mild tension for 20 to 30 seconds

Aerobic Exercise

Aerobic exercise is necessary to strengthen your heart, promote circulation, lower your glucose and blood pressure, and control weight by burning calories. Any activity that involves the use of the large muscles of the body simultaneously and elevates the heart rate can be considered aerobic. It needs to be sub-maximal in intensity and sustained for a minimum of 20 to 30 minutes. Walking, jogging, cycling, cross-country skiing, and step aerobics are all considered aerobic exercises suitable for diabetics. This book will feature aerobic exercises using a mini-trampoline. The aerobic exercises are also shown without a trampoline, so the choice is yours.

The recommendations of the American College of Sports Medicine's (ACSM) for aerobic training and conditioning for diabetics are as follows:

TYPE 1 DIABETES

Intensity: 60 to 90 percent maximum heart rate (MHR)
   (220- your age = MHR).
   Multiply MHR x .60 (60%) = low end of your target heart rate
Duration: 20 to 60 minutes with a 5 to 10 minute warm up and
   cool down
Frequency: Daily for better glucose control

TYPE 2 DIABETES

Intensity: 60 to 90 percent maximum heart rate
Duration: 20 to 60 minutes
Frequency: 3 to 5 times per week
Type of Activities: walking, jogging, cycling, stair climbing,
   cross-country skiing, swimming
Intensity: 60 to 90 percent maximum heart rate. Maximum heart
   rate can be calculated by subtracting your age from 220, and
   multiplying that number by the desired percentage. For example, a 40-year-old who is starting an aerobic exercise program
   and wishes to begin at the low end of their training heart rate
   (a wise decision), training heart rate would be:
   220 - 40 = 180 x .60 = 108

The target heart rate is 108 beats per minute. You can take your
pulse from the radial artery, just below the thumb, on your wrist.
Count your pulse for 10 seconds and multiply by 6. This will give
you your heart rate at that moment. Another way to monitor how
hard you are working is to pay attention to how you feel. The rate
of perceived exertion (RPE) is a numeric scale that is a subjective
measurement of how much you feel you are exerting yourself. You
rate yourself based on a scale of 6 to 20. An exertion level of 7 is
very, very light and a level of 19 is very, very, hard or a near maximal effort. You would not want to work at a level of 19. It is recom-

mended that you describe your effort as being fairly light to hard (11 to 15). This method is good to use if you have difficulty feeling your pulse or if you don't have a heart-rate monitor.

If you are out of condition and just starting to exercise, begin at low intensity, short duration, then progress to low intensity, long duration and then attempt to increase the intensity. Always begin with a low intensity warm up, which includes mild stretching, and finish with a cool down stretch. This will give you a smoother transition into exercise and reduces the possibility of muscle soreness or injury.

Duration: You should exercise for 20 to 60 minutes at your training heart rate. This does not include the warm up (10 to 15 minutes) or the cool-down (5 to 10 minutes)

Frequency: Daily exercise is recommended for insulin dependent diabetics for the best blood glucose control. Three to 5 times per week (or daily) is suggested for type 2, non-insulin dependent diabetics.

Strength Training

Strength training with weights increases lean muscle. This in turn, increases your metabolism and your calorie requirement at rest. Your goal is to increase muscle and decrease body fat to lower your insulin resistance. ACSM recommendations for strength training are as follows:

TYPE 1 AND TYPE 2 DIABETES

Resistance: moderate level using light weights (barbells and dumbells or machines)

Repetitions: 10 to 15 reps

Sets: 1 to 3

Frequency: 2 to 3 non-consecutive days per week

Select 8 to 10 exercises for the major muscles of the body

Strength training using light to moderate weights, or circuit training using resistance equipment is appropriate for diabetics. Keep repetitions between 10 and 15 reps. Include exercises for the major muscles of the body including the chest, upper back, abdomen, shoulders, buttocks, and thighs. You can also include strengthening exercises for the arms and calves.

You should take the exercise to the point of muscular fatigue, not failure, which is the inability to perform another repetition. When you can perform 15 reps with relative ease than you can increase the weights. Remember if you have high blood pressure you will need to keep the weights light and perform more repetitions. If you have uncontrolled hypertension than you should not lift weights, but you will need to discuss this with your doctor.

Exercise Recommendations for Diabetic Related Conditions

Retinopathy: You should avoid high intensity, strenuous exercise, or breath holding during exercise. Do not perform any exercise in which the head is down or lower than the body, for example, an incline sit up or bench press, or with some yoga positions. Instead of aerobics on the trampoline, choose the floor aerobic exercises. Consult with an ophthalmologist for additional guidelines and specific recommendations.

Autonomic Neuropathy: If you have type 2 diabetes avoid exercising in high temperatures due to the possibility of impaired regulation of body temperature. This will increase the likelihood of dehydration or hypothermia. You may be at greater risk for hypoglycemia and hypertension.

An elevated heart rate and lowered maximal heart rate can occur with autonomic neuropathy and will require you to use the perceived exertion method to keep track of intensity rather than heart rate.

Peripheral Neuropathy: Because of reduced sensation in your feet, diabetics with peripheral neuropathy should avoid exercise that could traumatize the feet such as prolonged hiking, or walking on uneven surfaces. You should select low- or non-impact exercises such as biking or swimming, which produce minimal jarring. It is important to check your feet daily for blisters and the general condition of your feet. Keep your feet warm and dry and practice good foot hygiene. Carefully choose sneakers and shoes for a proper fit. Make sure that the socks you are wearing fit properly over your feet without any folds.

Hypertension: You should avoid heavy weight lifting and breath holding, both of which could increase blood pressure. Use lighter weights with higher repetitions.

Precautions

You should have a medical checkup with the necessary testing by your doctor before beginning an exercise program. I suggest that you thoroughly review all exercises before you begin the program. Have a dress rehearsal of the exercises before you go full steam ahead. Be aware of the signs and symptoms of hypoglycemia (low blood sugar). Some of the symptoms such as sweating or high heart rate are also natural responses to exercise.

However, if you should feel dizzy, confused, have palpitations, tremors, or blurry vision, stop exercising and check your sugar levels. Be prepared to call 911. You should have a carbohydrate readily available every time you exercise. Make sure you have your cell phone or house phone nearby.

If you have autonomic neuropathy, use the exertion rating or talk test to monitor the intensity of your workout since your heart rate response may be blunted. Your blood pressure may also may be more sensitive to exercise and the ability of regulatory system to maintain appropriate body temperatures may be impaired. This can make you more prone to dehydration, so make sure you drink water before, during, and after exercise.

General Recommendations for Fluid Replacement: 17 to 20 oz 2 to 3 hours before exercise, 6 to 10 oz every 10 to 15 minutes during exercise for a total of 28 to 40 oz for every hour of exercise, and 6 to 10 oz after warm up. Replace lost fluid within 2 hours after exercise, 20 to 24 oz for every pound lost.

9

Aerobics Exercises

Aerobics is a fun way to shed some of those extra pounds. These exercises are designed to be done either on a mini-trampoline, or on the floor if a trampoline is not available or is considered unsafe for the exerciser.

Aerobics on the Mini-Trampoline

The mini-trampoline is a great aerobic training apparatus. It's fun, inexpensive, convenient and easily stored under a bed or in a closet. It can be purchased at most sporting goods stores. Jogging on a mini-trampoline is just as effective as jogging on a treadmill, without the impact and the stress on the joints. Not only is it a low-impact alternative to jogging or walking outdoors, which makes it ideal for diabetics, it also enhances balance. However, if you have peripheral neuropathy you should choose a non-weight-bearing aerobic exercise such as cycling or swimming.

Exercise tips for the mini-trampoline:

1. Keep your center of gravity low.
2. Push down as you jump, rather than jumping up, as you would on the ground.
3. Keep your knees slightly bent and lean slightly forward from the hip (not the spine). Keep your knees soft as you land.
4. The height of your bounce should be approximately 2 inches off the trampoline, so you will want to keep fairly close to the trampoline. This will give you better control with your movements.
5. Hold your abdominal muscles in and keep your pelvis tucked (neutral).
6. Wear supportive sneakers. Do not exercise wearing socks or with bare feet.
7. To inspire and motivate yourself, play your favorite music while you exercise.
8. Keep your posture erect, your head up and your focus forward. Hold your shoulders down and back with the chest open to allow the lungs to inflate adequately. Lift your rib cage up and away from the hips. Try not to sink into your body, but rather stay lifted. This will facilitate good breathing throughout the exercise.
9. Always keep your body centered in the middle of the trampoline. Keep all foot movements contained within the boundaries of the trampoline. Don't go overboard and step on the springs or the frame.

Aerobics on the Floor

While the mini-trampoline works for many people, it may not work for you. If you have poor balance, are not comfortable on the trampoline, or are very overweight, you may need to begin these exercises on the floor. This is slightly more high-impact but still very effective at burning fat.

The exercise tips for floor aerobics are as follows:

1. Hold your abdominal muscles in and keep your pelvis tucked (neutral).
2. Wear supportive sneakers. Do not exercise wearing socks or with bare feet.
3. To inspire and motivate yourself, play your favorite music while you exercise.
4. Keep your posture erect, your head up, and your focus forward. Hold your shoulders down and back, with the chest open to allow the lungs to inflate adequately. Lift your rib cage up and away from the hips. Try not to sink into your body, but rather stay lifted. This will facilitate good breathing throughout the exercise.

The Exercises

The following arm exercises are performed while stepping, marching, or jogging lightly on the trampoline or floor.

Front Raise

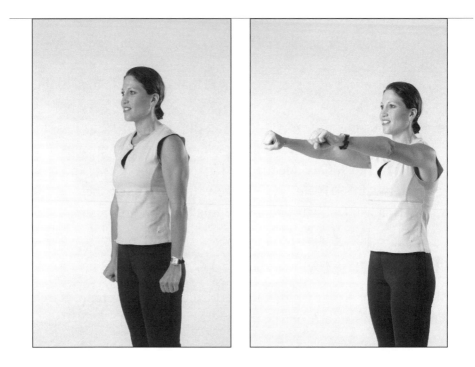

1 Hold arms at your sides with palms facing the rear.

2 Raise them to shoulder height and then lower them to your sides.

Variation: If your arms get tired you can lift and lower one arm at a time, alternating the right and left arm.

Side Raise

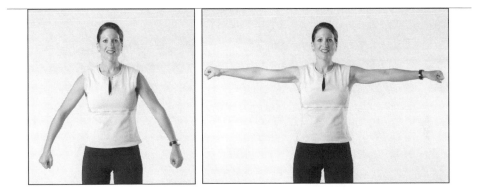

1. Raise your extended arms out to the sides to shoulder height.
2. Lower them to your sides.

Variation: If your arms get tired, you can lift and lower one arm at a time, alternating the right and left arms.

Front Crisscross

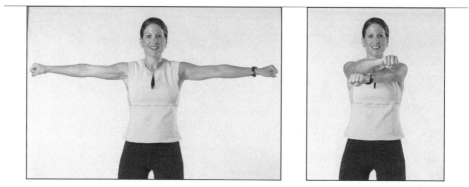

1 Start with your arms out to the sides.

2 Cross them to the front at chest level and return them to the sides.

3 Alternate crossing the right arm over the left and the left arm over the right.

Overhead Press

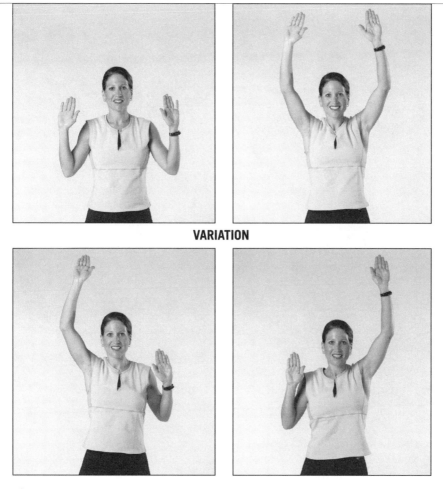

VARIATION

① Position your hands at your shoulders.
② Press both hands up and over your head.

Variation: If your arms get tired, you can lift and lower one arm at a time, alternating the right and left arms.

Front Press

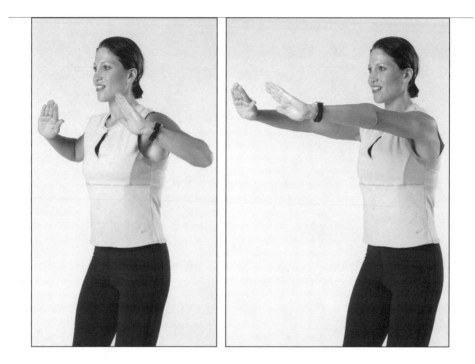

1. Position your hands at your shoulders.
2. Press your arms to the front at chest level.

Biceps Curl

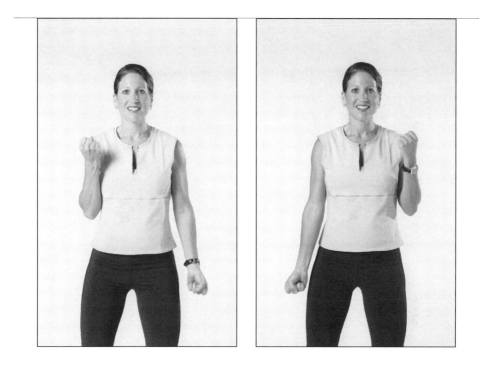

1 Bring your arms down to your sides.

2 Bend your elbows and curl you lower arms up so the hands come up to the shoulders.

3 Lower them back to the sides.

Low Rows

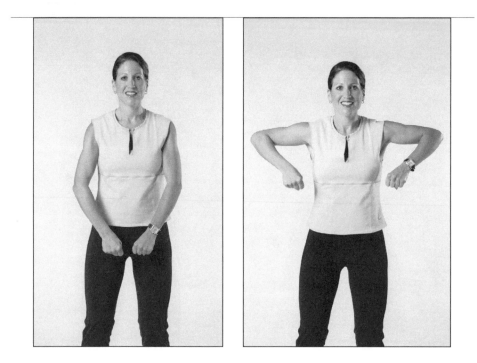

① Start with your arms down and fists together.
② Bend your elbows and pull your arms upward in a rowing motion. Let your elbows lead the movement. Do not lift your elbows higher than shoulder height.

Pullbacks

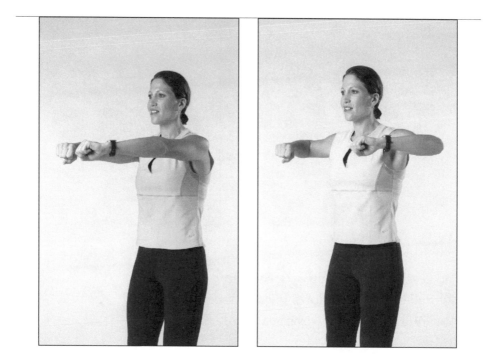

1 Extend your arms to the front and place your hands together at chest level.

2 Pull your elbows back, pinching your shoulder blades together.

3 Return the arms to the front.

Pulldowns

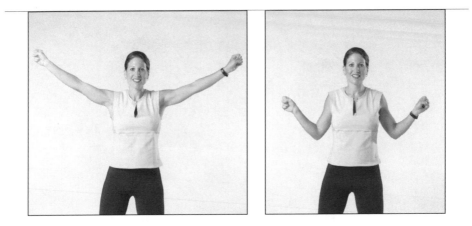

1 Reach both arms up over your head.
2 Pull both elbows down towards the rib cage.
3 Return them to the overhead position.

Tricep Press

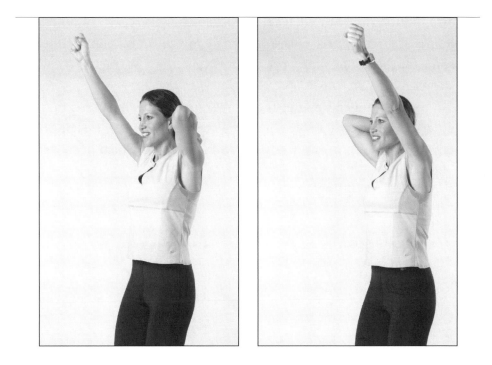

1. Keep both arms overhead. Alternating right and left arms, bend the elbows so your hand comes down to the shoulder.
2. Extend the elbow and press your hand away from the shoulder.

Aerobic Conditioning

After you have warmed up by jogging in place with the hand and arm motions as pictured, it's time to step your exercise up a notch. Some of these exercises are designed for the mini-trampoline, some for the floor. Some work for both, and these are pictured and starred.

You will notice some of the exercises are more strenuous than others. Be your own judge and decide according to your level of fitness what exercises you may want to include and which ones you may want to add on later.

Scissors

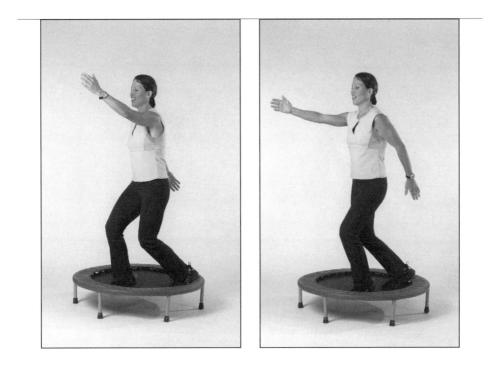

① Place your right foot in front of your left foot.

② Press away from the trampoline and switch your feet so the left is in front and the right is in back. Alternate, scissoring the right and left foot.

Low Kicks*

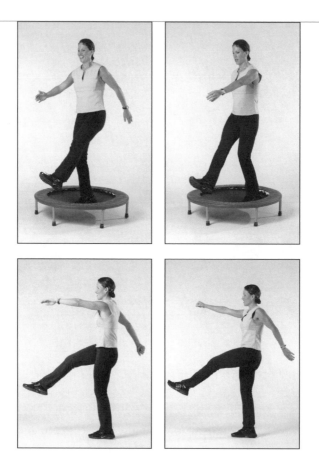

1 Step on your right foot and kick out your left foot low to the front. Then step on your left foot and kick out your right foot low to the front.

2 Let your arms swing, front to back, in opposition to your legs.

Skipping Rope

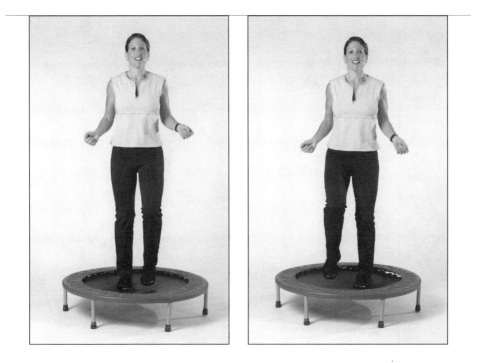

① Keeping your feet close to the trampoline, alternate lifting your feet.

② Circle your arms to the sides as if you were swinging a jump rope. Keep your elbows close to the sides.

Jump Rope*

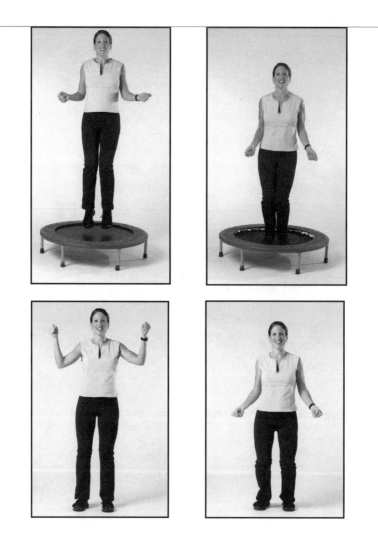

① Continue swinging your "jump rope."

② Instead of skipping, bounce with two feet at the same time. Keep your feet slightly apart, knees soft, and bounce lightly.

Jump Rope Wide*

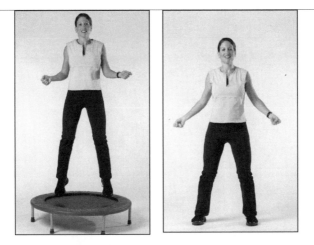

1. Continue swinging your "jump rope."
2. Instead of jumping with your feet together, keep them wide apart.

Jump Rope Narrow/Wide*

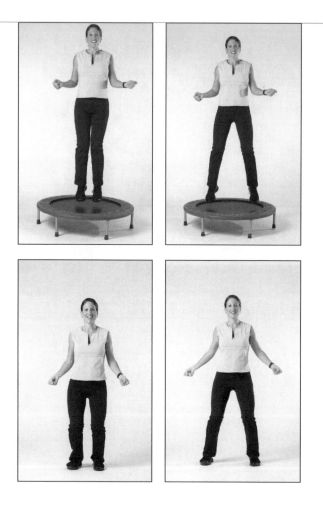

❶ Start with the feet together and bounce 4 times.

❷ Bounce your feet out wide and bounce 4 times. Again your arms will circle out to the sides as if you were swinging a jump rope.

Jumping Jacks

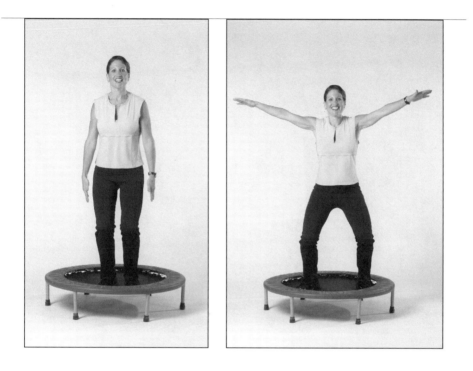

① Start with your feet together, in the center of the trampoline with your arms to your sides.

② Press away from the trampoline and jump your feet out. At the same time bring your arms out to the sides at shoulder height.

③ Bounce your feet back together and return the arms to your sides.

Slow Jacks

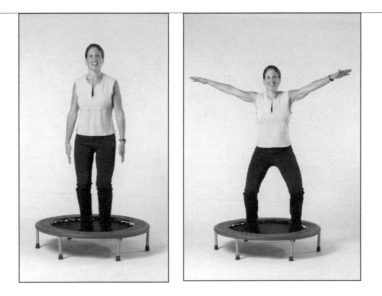

❶ Start in the center of the trampoline, with your feet together and your arms to your sides.

❷ Press away from the trampoline, jump your feet out, and bring your arms out to the sides at shoulder height.

❸ Bounce your feet back together, then bounce once more. Lower the arms to your sides.

Note: This exercise is just another version of the jumping jack, except that you take two little bounces with your feet together and two little bounces with your feet apart. In other words, the movement action will be: bounce in-in, bounce out-out. The arms will follow the same motion as the feet.

Knee Lifts*

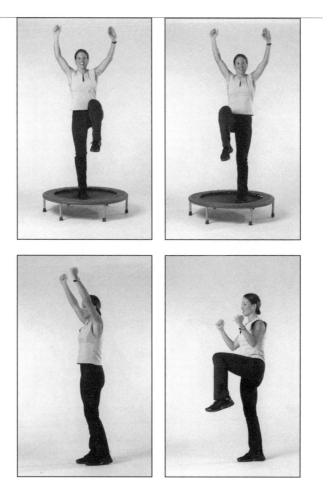

① Bounce with two feet, then lift your right knee up.

② Bounce with two feet and then lift your left knee up.

③ Alternate knee lifts right and left. The movement action will be: bounce-lift right bounce-lift left. Press your arms up as you lift each knee.

Knee Pump*

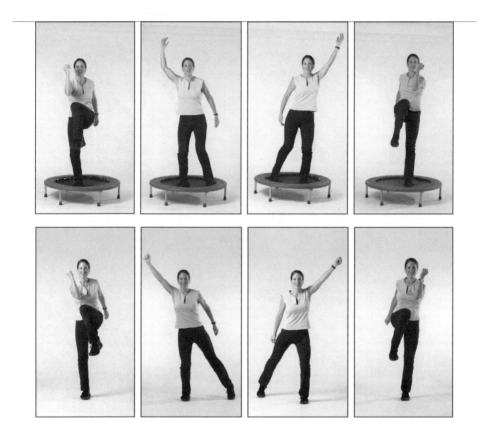

1 Bounce with two feet, then pump the right knee up and down 4 times as you pull the opposite elbow toward the knee.

2 Repeat the knee pumps on the left knee. Alternate the right and left knee pumps.

V-Step*

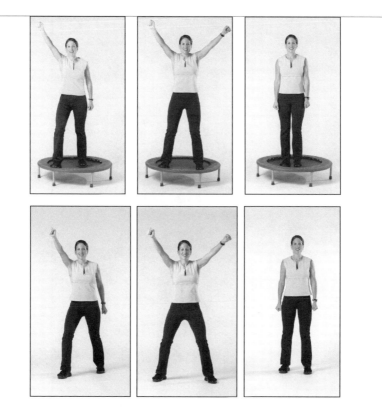

① Start with your feet together. Step your right foot out then step your left foot out in a V shape.

② Bounce and jump your feet back together.

③ Repeat with the left foot leading the movement. The movement action is step out-out, jump your feet back together. Your arms should follow the action of your feet.

Variation: To make it easier, perform the V-step with the right leg first 8 times, then repeat with the left leg 8 times.

Low Jog

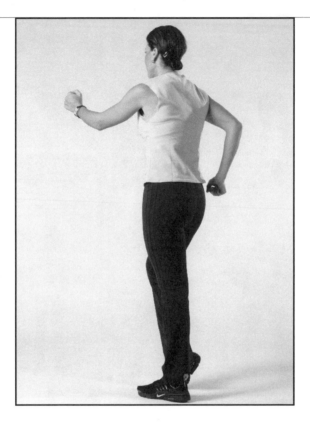

This is a low-impact version of a jog.

1 Your feet should be slightly apart. Instead of lifting your full foot off the ground, lift just the heel.

2 Alternate the heel lifts, keeping the balls of the feet in contact with the floor. If you don't have any joint problems or feel you need to work at a higher level you can lift the feet off the floor and jog in place, or you can march in place.

Low Skip Kicks

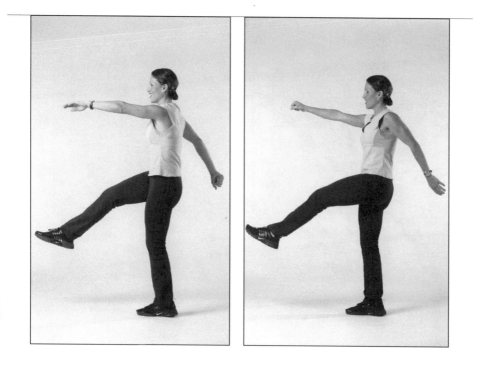

1 Step on your right foot and kick out your left foot low to the front, then step on your left foot and kick out your right foot low to the front.

2 Let your arms swing, front to back, in opposition to your legs. There should be a little bounce, or skip, between kicks when you transfer your weight from one foot to the other.

Half Jacks

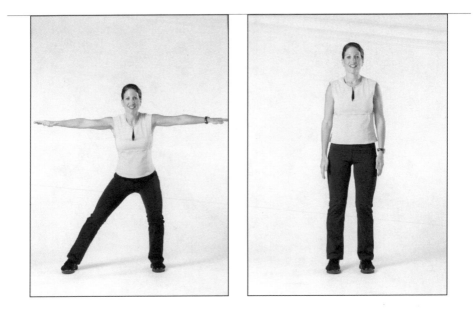

1. Start with your feet together, and your arms to your sides.
2. Step your right leg out to the side and squat down slightly. At the same time bring your arms out to the sides at shoulder height.
3. Push off from the floor with your right foot and bring your feet back together and return the arms back down to your sides.
4. Now step your left foot out, squat down slightly, push off and bring the feet together. Alternate half jacks right and left.

Tap Backs

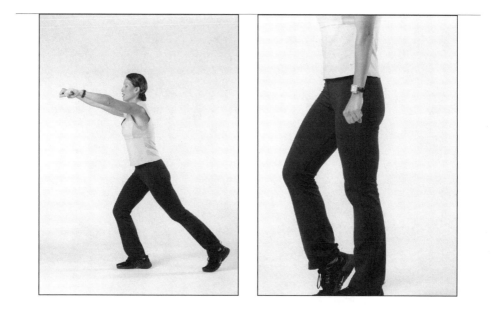

1 Start with your feet together.

2 Tap your right foot to the back and return it to center, tap your left foot back and return it to center.

3 Alternate tapping the right and left foot to the back as you press both arms to the front.

Hamstring Curls

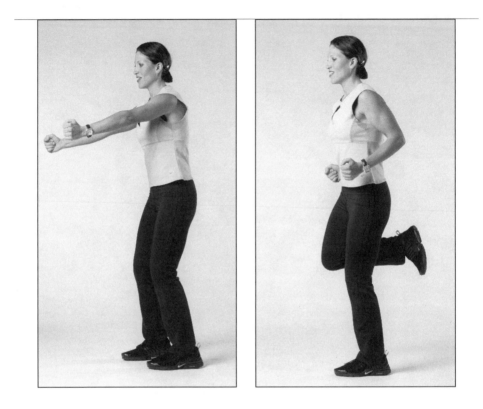

➊ Stand with your feet shoulder-width apart.

➋ Alternate lifting and lowering your right and lift foot to the back. Keep your knee directly under the hip as the knee bends and the heel moves towards the buttocks.

➌ Pull both arms back, in a low rowing motion, as you lift the heels.

Jab-Bob and Weave

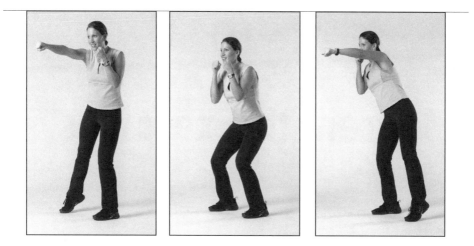

1 Stand with your feet wide.

2 Position your hands in front of your face with closed fists.

3 Squat down and swing your body to the right. As you come up, punch your left arm out to the front quickly and return it to the face.

4 Shift your body weight to your left leg, swing your body to the left, and punch with your right arm. Continue shifting (bob and weave) right and left as you punch with your left and right arm.

10

Strength Exercises

Research has shown that strengthening exercises are safe and effective for women and men of all ages, including those not in perfect health. In fact, people with health concerns—including heart disease or arthritis—often benefit the most from an exercise program that includes lifting weights a few times each week. Strength training, particularly in conjunction with regular aerobic exercise, can also have a profound impact on a person's mental and emotional health.

Strength training is just as important for diabetics as it is for the general population. Increasing muscle mass is important for good joint and muscle function, and it also boosts your metabolism. If you have more muscle, more calories are burned, which is an important consideration if you are interested in weight loss. Studies now show that lifestyle changes such as strength training have a profound impact on helping older adults manage their diabetes. In a recent study of Hispanic men and women, 16 weeks of strength training produced dramatic improvements in glucose control comparable to taking diabetes medication. Additionally, the study volunteers were stronger, gained muscle, lost body fat, had less depression, and felt much more self-confident.

Doing exercises with hand weights, elastic bands, or weight machines two or three times a week builds muscle. When you have more muscle and less fat, you'll burn more calories because muscle burns more than fat, even between exercise sessions. Strength training can help make daily chores easier, improve your balance and coordination, and strengthen your bones. You can strength train at home, at a fitness center, or in a class. Your health care team can tell you more about strength training and what kind is best for you.

Guidelines

The recommendation for resistance training is 2 to 3 non-consecutive days per week. The session should include at least one set of 8 to 10 exercises using all of the major muscles of the body. Each set of a strength exercise should consist of 8 to 15 repetitions. If you have hypertension or retinopathy, speak with your doctor before strength training. Diabetics with hypertension, joint problems, or mild retinopathy should keep the weights light and perform 12 to 15 repetitions of each exercise. Increase the weight only after you can easily perform 15 repetitions with proper form.

If you have never strength trained before, begin with body weight exercises. Don't use any weights, but allow the weight of your limb or body to be the resistance. When you feel ready, progress to free weights and/or resistance machines. As your strength improves you may perform a second or third set of each exercise; however, allow a 15 to 20 second rest period between sets.

Gather up, and have handy, all the supplies you'll need for your workout, such as: water bottle, glucose meter, exercise record book, towel, and a carbohydrate snack. You will also need a clock or watch to time each exercise.

Warm up before strength training, using the warm up from the aerobic section. Follow with the stretches given later in this book, in the flexibility section, after the strength session.

Technique

Strength exercises should be performed in a slow, controlled manner with good form and alignment. You should keep the joints soft and never lock out or fully extend them. Be careful to use the full range of motion. Don't grip the weights so tightly that your knuckles turn white. The most important thing is to breathe during the exercise. Exhale on the exertion phase and inhale on the preparatory phase of the exercise. If you hold your breath during exercise, particularly with strength training, you can drive your blood pressure up to dangerous levels. Choose a weight with which you can perform the exercise with good technique, that will allow you to feel tension within the muscle without strain.

The strength exercises in this section are basic and easy to follow, and cover the major muscles in the body. Perform 8 to 15 repetitions for each exercise. A sample workout program appears in Chapter 14.

Overhead Press

Target Area: Shoulder

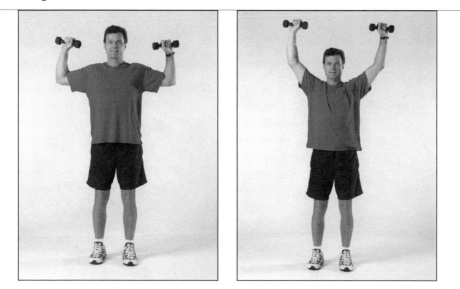

❶ Place your hands by your shoulders with your palms facing forward. Your hands should be slightly wider than your shoulders.

❷ Press your arms overhead without locking the elbow joint.

❸ Bring the weights together as you press upward and return the weights to the starting position. Your arms should be slightly in front of your head when you press up rather than directly over your head. Angling the arms slightly to the front will prevent injury to the shoulder. Keep your shoulders down and the spine in a neutral alignment (not arched) as you perform the exercise.

Variation: Single Arm Overhead Press. Alternate pressing the arms up overhead.

Lateral Raise

Target Area: Shoulder

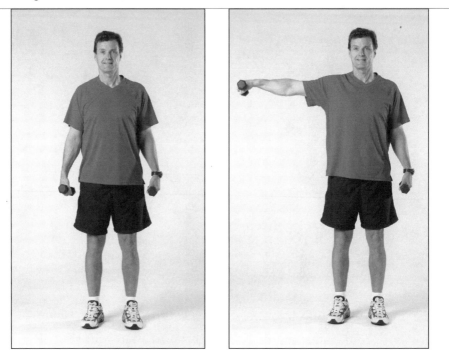

① Start with your arms at your sides and your feet shoulder width apart. Stand tall with your head in line with your spine. Keep your hips neutral.

② Raise your right arm to the side, up to shoulder height, pause at the top, and slowly lower the arm back down to your side.

③ Repeat with the left arm. Alternate lifting and lowering the right and left arms.

Note: Do not raise your arm above shoulder height.

Front Raise

Target Area: Front Shoulder

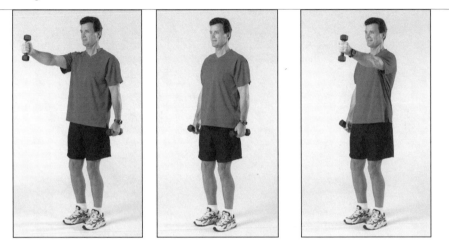

❶ Start with your arms at your sides and your feet shoulder width apart. Stand tall with your head in line with your spine. Keep your hips neutral.

❷ Raise your arms to the front, up to shoulder height, and slowly lower them back to your sides. Another option is to alternate lifting and lowering the right and left arm for 8 to 15 repetitions each.

Pullback

Target Area: Upper and Mid Back

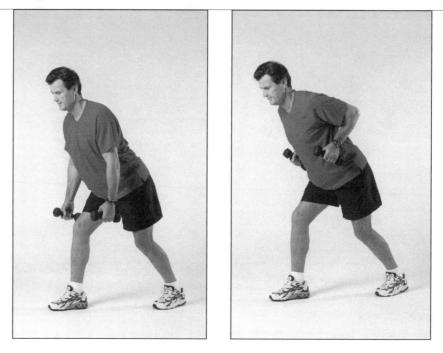

① Stand with one leg in front of the other. Balance your body weight between your legs and lean slightly forward from the hip.

② Bring both arms low, to the front.

③ Holding the weights with your palms facing each other, pull your elbows to the back, pinching your shoulder blades together, and then return to the starting position. Keep your shoulders down and your abdominal muscles contracted.

Biceps Curl

Target Area: Biceps

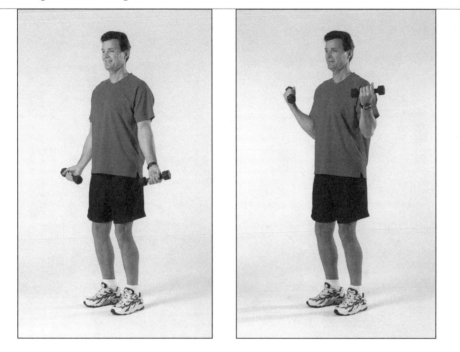

❶ Stand with your arms at your sides, palms forward and elbows soft.

❷ Slowly bend the elbows and lift the weight up towards the shoulder, pause at the top and then lower the weight to the starting position.

Squats

Target Area: Thigh and Buttocks

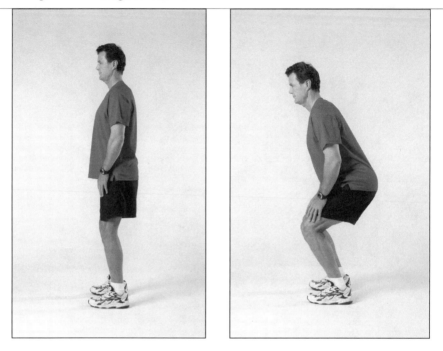

❶ Stand with your feet shoulder width apart. Place your body weight onto your heels and drop your hips to the back as you bend your knees.

❷ Slowly lower your hips as if you were sitting in a chair. Keep your abdominal muscles in and make sure you keep the knees behind the toes. If your knees come in front of the toes it can be stressful to the knees. Correct this by pushing your hips to the back. Also, be careful to not squat down too far. If your hips drop down below the knees then you are squatting too low.

Note: No weights are needed.

Hip Hiker

Target Area: Thigh and Buttocks

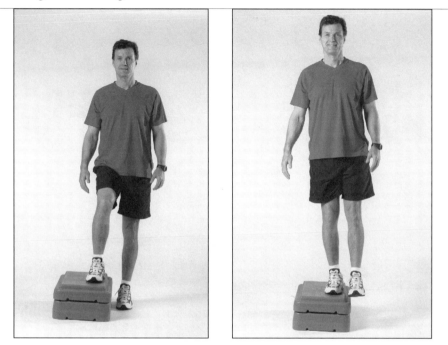

1. Stand to the side of the first step of your stairs.
2. Place the inside leg on top of the step.
3. Slowly straighten the knee and lift your opposite leg off the floor until it is level with the step.
4. Slowly lower the foot to the floor. Perform 8 to 15 repetitions, then repeat with the opposite leg.

Note: No weights are needed.

STRENGTH EXERCISES PERFORMED WHILE SUPINE

Chest Press

Target Area: Chest, Pectorals

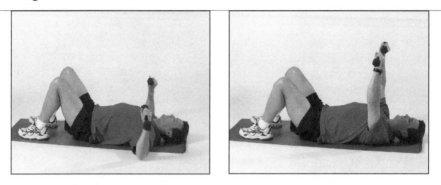

1 Lie on your back with your knees bent and feet in contact with the floor.

2 Bring your elbows out to the sides and position your lower arms and hands directly over your elbows.

3 Press the weights toward the ceiling, extending your arms without locking your elbows. Keep your wrists in a straight line. Slowly lower to the starting position.

Flies

Target Area: Chest, Pectorals

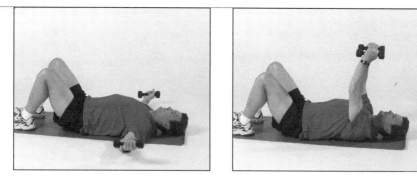

1 Place yours arms out to the sides at chest level. Your hands should be lower than the shoulder joint.

2 Bring both arms up over your chest. You should feel the tension in the chest muscles as you bring the weights together up over your chest.

3 Slowly lower the weights to the starting position. Remember to keep the elbows soft as you perform the exercise.

Triceps Extensions

Target Area: Triceps

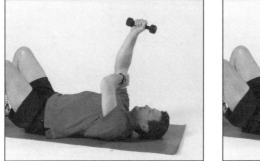 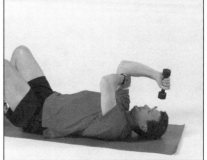

1 Hold a weight in your right hand.

2 Place your extended right arm directly over the right shoulder. Support the right elbow with left hand.

3 Bring your right hand down toward the right shoulder and then press it back up to the extended position.

Variation: Cross-Over Triceps Extensions

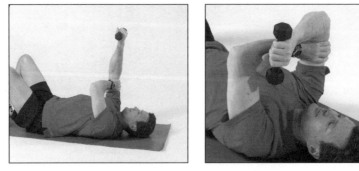

Target Area: Triceps

1 Placing your extended right arm directly in line with your right shoulder. Use your left hand to support the right elbow.

2 Next, instead of lowering the weight to your right shoulder, lower it toward your left shoulder and then press it back up to the extended position.

Abdominal Curl-Ups

Target Area: Abdominals

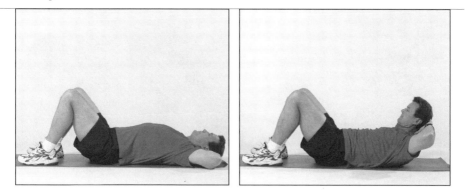

1 Lie flat on the floor with your knees bent and your feet in contact with the floor. Support your head by placing your hands at the base of your head.

2 Without pressing your head forward, slowly lift your head, neck, and shoulders up away from the floor. Press your back toward the floor as you lift. Lift to the point at which your shoulders and upper back come up away from the floor. Engage the abdominal muscles and exhale as you lift.

3 Pause at the top of the lift and then slowly lower the upper back, shoulders, neck, and head to the floor.

Note: No weights are needed.

Core Stabilization

Target Area: Torso

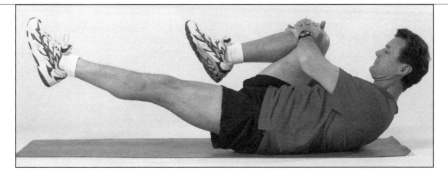

● Lie flat on the floor.

● Bring one knee in towards your chest.

● Lift your head, neck, and shoulders, as one unit, up toward the knee. Contract the abdominals as you hold the position. Allow the contraction of the torso muscles to hold you up rather than the arms. Count to 8.

● Switch your legs so the left knee is bent and the right leg is straight. Keep your upper body lifted as you switch legs. Count to 8, then switch legs again.

● Repeat with the right leg, holding for a 4 count, switch legs hold for a 4 count on the left.

● Switch to the right and hold for a 2 count, then hold for a 2 count on the left.

● Finish with a single count, switching the right and left knee for 8 counts while your upper body stays lifted away from the floor. Keep your abdominals contracted for the duration of the exercise. Don't forget to breathe while you hold the contraction. Holding your breath during exercise can be dangerous.

Note: No weights are needed.

Crossover Crunch

Target Area: Obliques

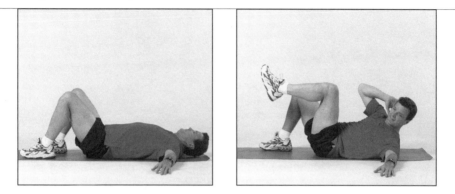

① Lie on your back with your knees bent and your feet a comfortable distance from your hips. Your spine should be pressed towards the floor.

② Place your right hand behind your head to provide support to the neck. Place your opposite arm out to the side.

③ Slowly lift your right shoulder up off the floor. As you lift the right shoulder, bring your left knee in toward your right elbow. Your right elbow crosses over to reach for the left knee. It is not important to actually touch the knee but the emphasis should be on the rotation of the spine. This will engage the obliques (waist muscles).

④ Slowly lower the right shoulder and at the same time extend the left leg out. Repeat crossing over the right elbow to the left knee. Repeat the exercise with the left elbow crossing over to the right knee.

Note: No weights are needed.

Side Leg Lifts

Target Area: Outer thigh/hip

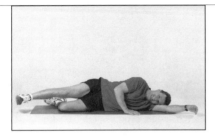 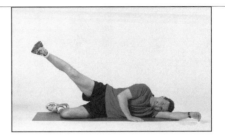

1 Lie on your side with your head resting on your arm. Stack your shoulders one on top of the other. Stack you hips so the top hip is directly over the bottom hip.

2 Place your top arm in front of your chest to support the body and prevent it from rocking front or back.

3 Bend your bottom leg and extend the top leg straight down.

4 Lift the top leg to hip height and then return the leg to the starting position.

Note: No weights are needed, but light ankle weights can be used after you can complete 15 reps comfortably. Start with 1 to 3 pound ankle weights.

Inner Thigh Lifts

Target Area: Inner Thighs

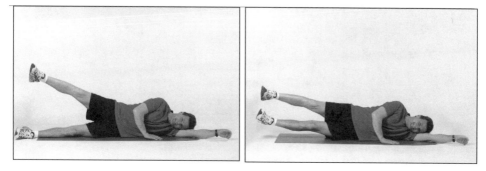

1 Lie on your side with your head resting on your arm. Stack your shoulders one on top of the other. Stack your hips so the top hip is directly over the bottom hip. Extend both legs straight down.

2 Place your top arm in front of your chest to support the body and prevent it from rocking front or back.

3 Lift your top leg up away from the floor and hold it up at approximately hip height.

4 Lift your extended lower leg up toward the top leg as if you were clapping your feet. Lift and lower your bottom leg. Repeat with the opposite leg.

Note: No weights are needed, but light ankle weights can be used after you can complete 15 reps comfortably. Start with 1 to 3 pound ankle weights.

Back Leg Lifts

Target Area: Buttocks and Hamstring

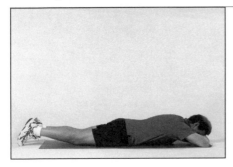 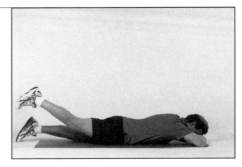

1 Lie facedown with your forehead resting on your hands.

2 Lift your right leg a few inches away from the floor. Keep your knee straight as you lift the leg and keep your hips in contact with the floor. Lift and lower your right leg and repeat on the left.

Note: No weights are needed, but light ankle weights can be used after you can complete 15 reps comfortably. Start with 1 to 3 pound ankle weights.

Modified Push-Ups

Target Area: Chest/Arms

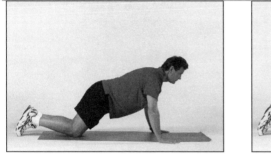 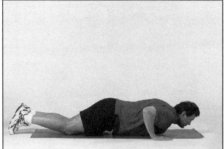

1 Position yourself on all fours (knees and hands) with your knees directly under or slightly behind your hips and your hands under you shoulders. Your back should be in a flat "table top" position. Keep your abdominal muscles contracted.

2 Slowly bend your elbows and lower your chest towards the floor.

3 Press away from the floor, straightening the elbows as you come back up to the starting position. Don't lock the elbows—keep them a little soft when you return to the starting position. Inhale on the way down and exhale as you come up.

Note: No weights are needed.

Shoulder Extensions

Target Area: Posterior shoulder

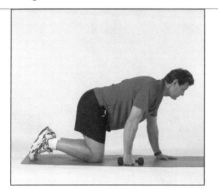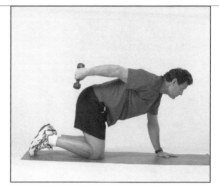

1 Position yourself on all fours (knees and hands) with your knees directly under your hips and your hands under you shoulders. Your back should be in a flat "table top" position. Keep your abdominal muscles contracted.

2 Hold a weight in your right hand.

3 Keep your right arm straight and lift it to the back. Hold it at the point when it is parallel to the floor.

4 Slowly lower the arm back down. Maintain the flat table top position, with your abdominals held in, as you perform this exercise. Lift and lower the right arm and repeat on the left.

11

Flexibility Training, Warm Ups, and Cool-Downs

Flexibility Training and Stretches

To make your fitness program complete you'll need to include regular sessions of flexibility training. The ideal time for flexibility training is after your workout since your muscles are warm and will respond better to stretching. Muscles are more pliable when they are warm because of the increased blood flow during exercise.

There is a difference between the stretches that are done in your warm up and the stretches that are performed after your workout. The purpose of the stretches that are done in your warm up is to prepare the muscles and joints for the workout and to possibly prevent injury. They are held for a shorter length of time (8 to 10 seconds). The stretches that you'll do at the end of your workout will increase flexibility and possibly prevent muscle soreness and cramping. These stretches are held longer (20 to 30 seconds).

As we age, we lose flexibility due to postural habits or inactivity. As a result, the tendons and muscles are not being put through their full range of motion. Eventually, this leads to muscle tightening. Any imbalance in muscle flexibility can bring about postural changes and misalignment. Flexibility training can counteract these changes.

Benefits of Flexibility Training

- Improved range of motion
- Decrease chance of injury
- Decreased muscle soreness associated with muscle use
- Improved posture
- Improved coordination

Technique

To realize the benefits of stretching you will need to follow a few guidelines:

1. Always stretch after the muscles are warmed up. A simple march for 3 minutes while you pump your arms will get your blood flowing to your muscles and increase muscle temperature.
2. Slowly ease your body into the stretch. Don't force the stretch. Take the stretch to the point of mild tension.
3. Never bounce as you stretch. This can cause the muscle to tighten and is counterproductive. Hold the stretch for 20 to 30 seconds and release. You can repeat the stretch if you want to.
4. Remember to breathe fully as you stretch. Don't hold your breathe. Slow, deep breathing will help you relax your muscles which will facilitate the stretch.

The stretches in this chapter target all your muscles, from head to toe. Stretching is a very safe activity and can be performed every day. It will help relieve stress and tension within your muscles.

Neck Stretch

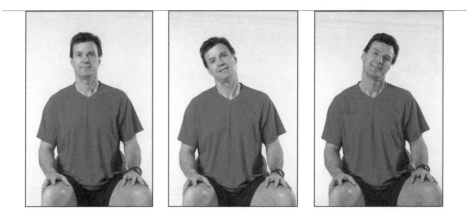

1 Sit comfortably in a chair, with your back supported and your fet flat on the floor.

2 Slowly drop your head to the side so your right ear moves towards the right shoulder. Keep your shoulders down and relaxed.

3 Holding the stretch, slowly bring the head back to center

4 Repeat on the opposite side.

Upper Trapezius Stretch

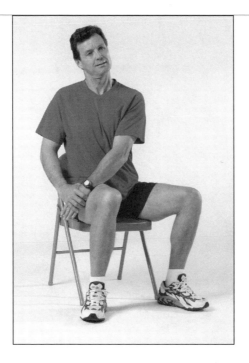

① Sit comfortably in a chair.

② Place your left hand across your lap onto your outer right thigh. Grab your left wrist with your right hand and apply a gentle downward pressure.

③ Drop your head to the right and hold the stretch.

④ Repeat the stretch on the opposite side.

Shoulder Stretch

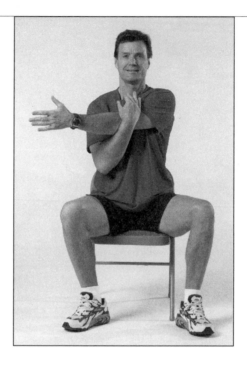

① Sit comfortably in a chair.

② Raise your arm to shoulder height, across your chest. Slightly bend the elbow. Gently pull your arm toward the front of your body with the opposite arm. Keep both shoulders down and relaxed. You should feel the stretch along the back of your shoulder.

③ Repeat the stretch on the opposite side.

Seated Side Bend Stretch

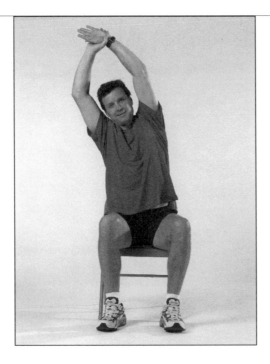

❶ Bring both arms overhead.

❷ Clasp your left wrist with your right hand and bend your upper body to the right side. Gently pull your left arm toward the right. Keep your hips in a neutral position. Hold the stretch and then relax the arms to your sides.

❸ Repeat on the opposite side, switching hand positions.

Chest Stretch

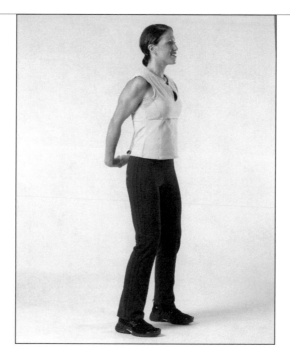

1 Clasp both hands behind your back.

2 Gently lift them up and away from your body. Keep your shoulders down as you hold the stretch.

Corner Chest Stretch

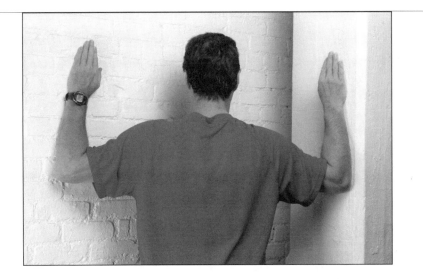

1 Stand facing a corner.

2 Raise your arms out to the sides with the elbows bent at a 90-degree angle, at shoulder height. Place one foot in front of the other.

3 Keep your head up as you lean your body forward. Press your chest through your arms.

Cat and Camel Stretch

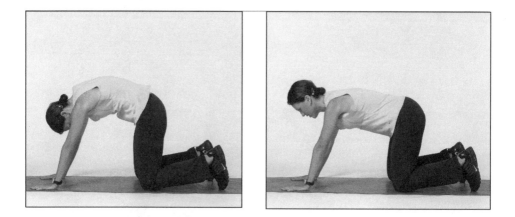

1 Kneel on all fours. Place your hands directly under your shoulders and your knees under your hips.

2 Arch your back toward the ceiling, rounding your back.

3 Hold this stretch 10 seconds and then release to a flat back. Repeat the stretch 3 to 5 times.

Knee to Chest Stretch

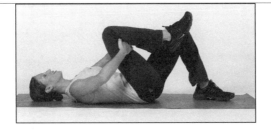

1 Lie on your back with both knees bent and the feet in contact with the floor.

2 Lift one knee in toward your chest. Clasp both hands behind the lifted knee and gently pull it in toward the chest.

3 Hold the stretch and repeat on the opposite leg. You should feel the stretch in the lower back, the buttock, and the back of the thigh.

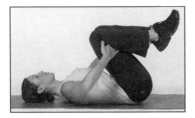

Variation: Double Knee to Chest Stretch

1 Lie on your back with both knees bent and the feet in contact with the floor.

2 Lift both knees in toward your chest. Clasp both hands behind the knees and gently pull them toward the chest.

3 Hold the stretch. You should feel the stretch in the lower back and buttocks, and the back of the thighs.

Back Rotation Stretch

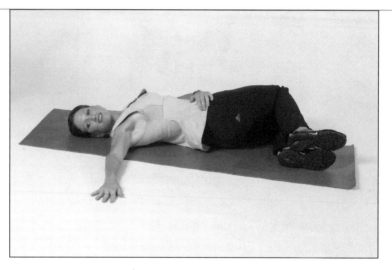

1 After completing the double knee stretch slowly drop both knees to the right side.

2 Let your arms reach out to the opposite side and turn your head in the direction of your arms.

3 Holding the stretch, slowly bring your knees to the center and then gradually drop them to the opposite side. Again the arms reach out in the opposite direction.

Hamstring Towel Stretch

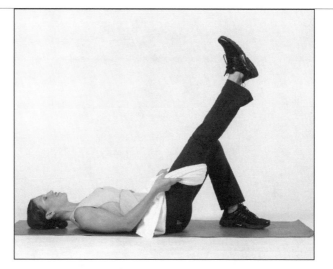

1 Lie on your back with one knee bent and the other extended up toward the ceiling.

2 Wrap a towel around the extended leg. Grab both ends and pull your leg gently toward you. You should feel the stretch in the back of your legs. Be careful not to overstretch the muscle.

3 Take it to the point of mild tension, hold, and then release.

4 Repeat on the opposite leg.

Inner Thigh Stretch

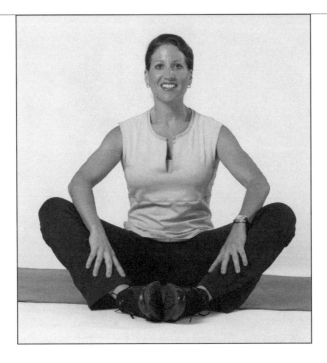

1 Sit on the floor with your back straight. Bring your feet together in front with your soles facing each other.

2 Place your forearms on your inner thighs and gently press your thighs down toward the floor.

Kneeling Stretch

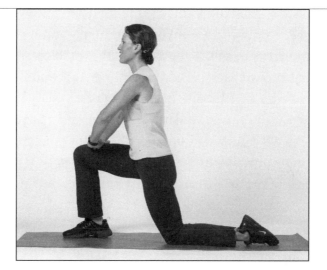

1 Start in a kneeling position. Bring your right leg to the front.

2 Rest your hands on your right thigh and press your body weight forward. You should feel the stretch in the front of your left hip and thigh. Make sure you right knee stays behind your toes. If you need to increase the stretch, slide your left leg back.

3 Hold the stretch and repeat the stretch on the opposite side.

Warm Ups

It is important to warm up before you start your workout. This will prepare your muscles and joints for the more strenuous exercises to follow. It will also reduce your chance of injury and lessen the possibility of muscle soreness. Keep in mind that mild soreness is a natural consequence of exercise when you first start training. You may be using muscles that haven't been active in a while. If the muscle soreness extends beyond two days it may indicate that you are overdoing it. Extend your warm up and stretch for your next workout and reduce the intensity of the strength training a bit.

A typical warm up will last 12 to 15 minutes. At this point, you are advised to check your pulse, drink a sip of water, and check your glucose.

You can record your numbers in the exercise log book. Include your rating, using the exertion scale, in the log book. It is important to keep moving by lightly stepping in place as you take your pulse and glucose, to avoid blood pooling in the lower legs. Stopping abruptly during exercising can cause dizziness or fainting.

WARM UP MOVEMENTS

Toe Taps

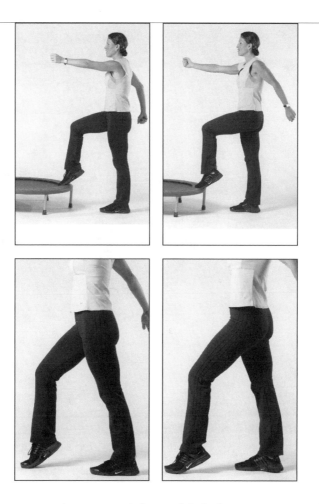

① Alternate tapping your right and left foot as you reach your arms in opposition to your feet.

② As your right foot taps, your left arm reaches forward. As your left foot taps up, your right arm reaches forward.

Runner's Lunge

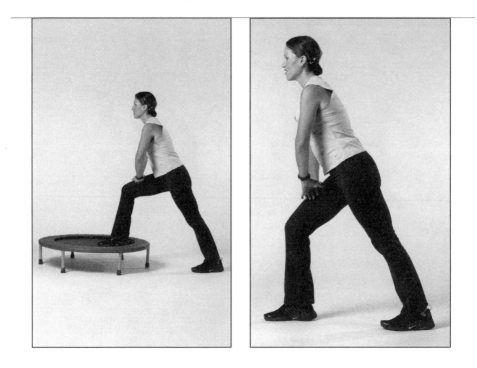

❶ Place your right foot in front of you.

❷ Bend your right knee and gently press your body weight forward onto the front leg. The left leg is extended behind you with the heel in contact with the floor. Make sure your right knee does not extend past your toes.

❸ Keep the knee at approximately 90 degrees. Support your upper body by placing your hands on the right thigh. You should feel this stretch in your left calf and the front of your left hip.

Calf Raises

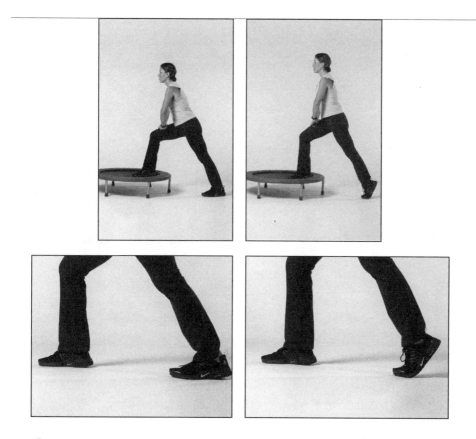

1 In the position of the Runner's Lunge, lift and lower the left heel 8 to 10 times.

Hamstring Stretch

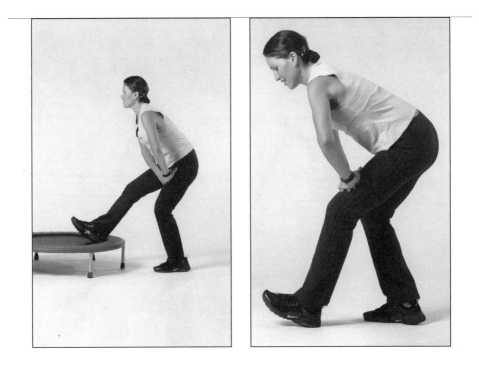

1 Shift your body weight onto your back leg. Place your right heel in front of you with the toes pointing towards the ceiling.

2 Press your hips to the back as you lean forward. Keep your hands supported on your thighs. Keep your knees soft, not locked. You should feel the stretch along the back of your leg.

3 Hold the stretch for 10 seconds.

Back Stretch

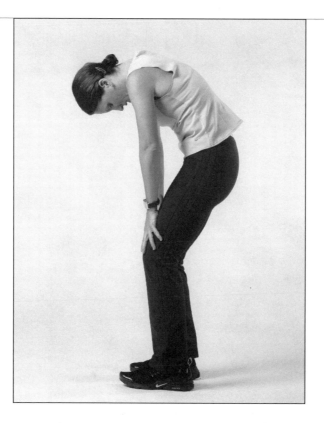

1 Place both hands on your thighs and bend your knees slightly, keeping your feet shoulder width apart.

2 Round your back and tuck your pelvis under. Hold the stretch for 10 seconds.

Step Marches

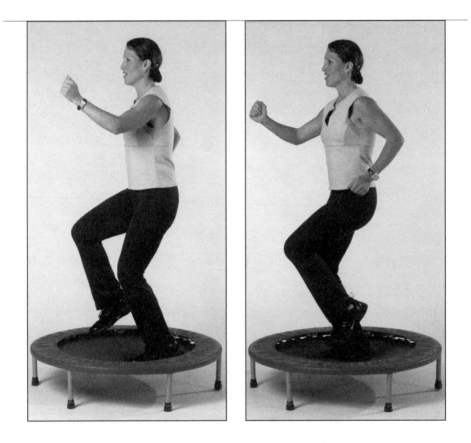

❶ Step up onto the center of the trampoline. Begin stepping in place, pumping your arms as you step. Lift your feet about 2 to 3 inches.

❷ As you continue through the warm up, gradually progress to a march. Increase the range of motion of your legs and arms. Lift your feet a little higher and and make your arm pumps bigger.

Cool-Downs

Equally important to an exercise regime is its cool-down period. It's never a good idea to simply stop a vigorous exercise and walk away. While cooling down, remember to check and record your blood glucose levels every 15 minutes. Fruit or another readily absorbed carbohydrate should be at hand.

Cool-down stretches differ from warm up stretches because you can hold them statically. Static stretches are held for 20 to 30 seconds and improve flexibility and ultimately increase the resting length of the muscle. This improvement in flexibility is yet another reason to take your time in the cool-down phase.

Step Touches

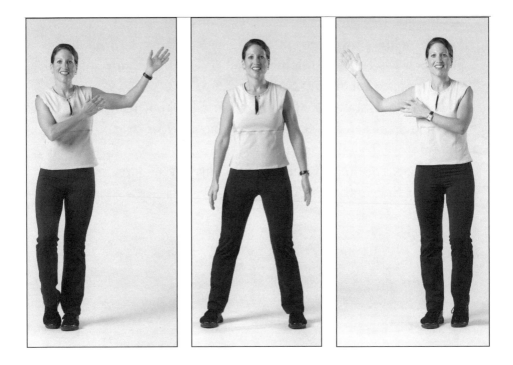

❶ Stay on top of the trampoline. Step your right foot out to the side, then bring the left foot in toward the right.

❷ Step your left foot out to the side and then close the right foot in toward the left foot. The action is step-together, step-together.

❸ Let your arms swing low right and left following the motion of your feet. Continue for 2 minutes.

❹ Step off the trampoline and continue the step touches on the floor for 1 minute.

Shoulder Stretch

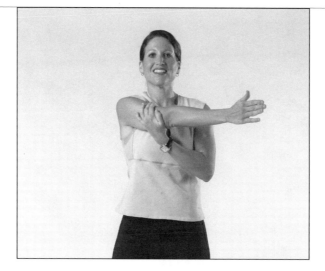

① Place your right arm across your chest.

② Place your left hand above your right elbow and gently press your elbow towards your right shoulder.

③ Repeat the stretch to the opposite shoulder.

Part III: The Workout

12

The Mini-Trampoline Aerobics Program

The following sample exercise program is a general guideline for you to follow. It is important to progress slowly when you begin to exercise, even though you may be very enthusiastic and want to do more. Listen to your body. If an exercise doesn't feel comfortable, then omit that particular exercise. Keep a log book on how hard you feel you are working, your heart rate, glucose levels, and any other information that you feel is important. A sample exercise log sheet is given on page 181. You can use the following exertion rating scale to describe how hard you feel you are working.

1   no effort, resting
2   very, very light
3   light
4   fairly light
5   somewhat hard
6   hard
7   very hard
8   very, very hard
9   near maximal effort
10 maximal effort

You should work at a rating of 4 to 6.

Pay attention to your breathing rate. This will also give you an indication that you might be working too hard. You should be able to breath freely and fully as you exercise. If you are panting as you try to catch your breath then you are working too hard and should lighten up a little. The talk test is a commonly used method of determining appropriate intensity. If you can talk comfortably as you exercise, then your exertion rate is OK.

When following this warm up program, make sure to follow the guidelines and instructions found in Chapter 11.

Tips for Staying Active

If the aerobic exercises in these workouts don't appeal to you or if you get bored of them, you can try alternating them with other aerobic exercise, such as:

- Hiking
- Climbing stairs
- Swimming or taking a water-aerobics class
- Dancing
- Playing basketball, volleyball, or other sports
- In-line skating, ice skating, or skate boarding
- Playing tennis
- Cross-country skiing

In addition, try to be extra active during the day. There are many ways to be extra active:

- Walk around while you talk on the phone
- Play with the kids
- Take the dog for a walk
- Get up to change the TV channel instead of using the remote control
- Work in the garden or rake leaves
- Clean the house
- Wash the car
- Park at the far end of the shopping center lot and walk to the store
- At the grocery store, walk down every aisle
- At work, walk over to see a co-worker instead of calling or emailing
- Take the stairs instead of the elevator
- Stretch or walk around instead of taking a coffee break and eating
- During your lunch break, walk to the post office or do other errands

SAMPLE MINI-TRAMPOLINE PROGRAM

WEEKS 1 TO 3

3x per week: **Monday/Wednesday/Friday or**

Tuesday/Thursday/Saturday or Sunday

WARM UP:

Begin by leading with the right leg.

March in place	1 minute
Toe Taps	2 minutes
Runner's Lunge	hold the stretch 10 seconds
Calf Raises	8x
Hamstring Stretch	hold 10 seconds
Back Stretch	hold 10 seconds
Step Marches	2 minutes
Low Jog	1 minute

Repeat the warm up exercise sequence with the left leg leading the movement.

TOTAL TIME 13 MINUTES

Check and record your pulse, glucose, and exertion rating. Drink 6 oz of water.

AEROBICS:

Step up onto the center of the mini-trampoline. Lift your feet about 2 to 3 inches. Gradually progress to a march, lifting your feet higher and making arm pumps bigger. Pick up the pace to a light jog while performing the following arm movements for one minute each.

Front Raise	Biceps Curl
Side Raise	Low Rows
Front Crisscross	Pullbacks
Overhead Press	Pulldowns
Front Press	Tricep Press

Continuing to jog, check your pulse and glucose, and record your exertion level. Drink 6 oz of water. Then perform the following trampoline exercises for 1 minute each.

Scissors	Jumping Jacks
Skipping Rope	Slow Jacks
Jump Rope	Knee Lifts
Jump Rope Wide	

TOTAL TIME APPROXIMATELY 17 MINUTES

COOL-DOWN:

Step Touches on the trampoline	2 minutes
Step Touches on the floor	1 minute
Runner's Lunge	
right leg	hold 20 seconds
left leg	hold 20 seconds
Hamstring Stretch	
right leg	hold 20 seconds
left leg	hold 20 seconds
Shoulder Stretch	
right shoulder	hold 20 seconds
left shoulder	hold 20 seconds
Chest Stretch	20 seconds

TOTAL TIME APPROXIMATELY 6 MINUTES

TOTAL EXERCISE SESSION TIME APPROXIMATELY 36 MINUTES

Check and record your pulse, glucose, and exertion rating. Drink 6 oz of water.

WEEKS 4 TO 6

3x per week: **Monday/Wednesday/Friday or**
Tuesday/Thursday/Saturday or Sunday

WARM UP:

Begin by leading with the right leg.

March in place	1 minute
Toe Taps	2 minutes
Runner's Lunge	hold the stretch 10 seconds
Calf Raises	10x
Hamstring Stretch	hold 10 seconds
Back Stretch	hold 10 seconds
Step Marches	2 minutes
Low Jog	2 minutes

Repeat the warm up exercise sequence with the left leg leading the movement.

TOTAL TIME 15 MINUTES

Check and record your pulse, glucose, and exertion rating. Drink 6 oz of water.

AEROBICS:

Step up onto the center of the mini-trampoline. Lift your feet about 2 to 3 inches. Gradually progress to a march, lifting your feet higher and making arm pumps bigger. Pick up the pace to a light jog, while performing the following arm movements for one minute each.

Front Raise	Biceps Curl
Side Raise	Low Rows
Front Crisscross	Pullbacks
Overhead Press	Pulldowns
Front Press	Tricep Press

Continuing to jog, check your pulse, glucose, and record your exertion level. Drink 6 oz of water. Then perform the following trampoline exercises for 1 minute each.

Scissors	Jumping Jacks
Low Kicks	Slow Jacks
Skipping Rope	Knee Lifts
Jump Rope	Knee Pump
Jump Rope Wide	V-Step
Jump Rope Narrow/Wide	

TOTAL TIME APPROXIMATELY 21 MINUTES

COOL-DOWN:

Step Touches on the trampoline	2 minutes
Step Touches on the floor	1 minute
Runner's Lunge	
right leg	hold 20 seconds
left leg	hold 20 seconds
Hamstring Stretch	
right leg	hold 20 seconds
left leg	hold 20 seconds
Shoulder Stretch	
right shoulder	hold 20 seconds
left shoulder	hold 20 seconds
Chest Stretch	20 seconds

TOTAL TIME APPROXIMATELY 6 MINUTES

TOTAL EXERCISE SESSION TIME APPROXIMATELY 42 MINUTES

Check and record your pulse and glucose, and exertion rating. Drink 6 oz of water.

WEEKS 7 TO 9

Follow the program from Weeks 4 to 6 but add an extra day of aerobic exercise per week. For example:

Monday/Wednesday/Friday/Saturday or Sunday

Tuesday/Thursday/Saturday/Sunday

WEEKS 10 TO 12

3x per week: **Monday/Wednesday/Friday or**

Tuesday/Thursday/Saturday or Sunday

WARM UP:

Begin by leading with the right leg

March in place	1 minute
Toe Taps	2 minutes
Runner's Lunge	hold the stretch 10 seconds
Calf Raises	10x
Hamstring Stretch	hold 10 seconds
Back Stretch	hold 10 seconds
Step Marches	2 minutes
Low Jog	2 minutes

Repeat the warm up exercise sequence with the left leg leading the movement.

TOTAL TIME 15 MINUTES

Check and record your pulse and glucose, and exertion rating. Drink 6 oz of water.

AEROBICS:

Step up onto the center of the mini-trampoline. Lift your feet about 2 to 3 inches. Gradually progress to a march, lifting your feet higher and making arm pumps bigger. Pick up the pace to a light jog while performing the following arm movements for 1 1/2 minutes each.

Front Raise	Biceps Curl
Side Raise	Low Rows
Front Crisscross	Pullbacks
Overhead Press	Pulldowns
Front Press	Tricep Press

Continuing to jog, check your pulse and glucose, and record your exertion level. Drink 6 oz of water. Then perform the following trampoline exercises for 1 minute each.

Scissors	Jumping Jacks
Low Kicks	Slow Jacks
Skipping Rope	Knee Lifts
Jump Rope	Knee Pump
Jump Rope Wide	V-Step
Jump Rope Narrow/Wide	

TOTAL TIME APPROXIMATELY 26 MINUTES

COOL-DOWN:

Step Touches on the trampoline	2 minutes
Step Touches on the floor	1 minute
Runner's Lunge	
right leg	hold 30 seconds
left leg	hold 30 seconds
Hamstring Stretch	
right leg	hold 30 seconds
left leg	hold 30 seconds
Shoulder Stretch	
right shoulder	hold 30 seconds
left shoulder	hold 30 seconds
Chest Stretch	30 seconds

TOTAL TIME APPROXIMATELY 7 MINUTES

TOTAL EXERCISE SESSION TIME APPROXIMATELY 48 MINUTES

Check and record your pulse and glucose, and exertion rating. Drink 6 oz of water.

WEEKS 12+

Follow the program from weeks 10 to 12 but perform all of the mini-trampoline exercises for 1 1/2 minutes. This will increase the length of time of the aerobic portion of your workout by 5 1/2 minutes. Your total exercise time will be approximately 53 1/2 minutes.

13

The Floor Aerobics Program

Floor Aerobics

The following aerobic exercises will get you up and moving. They are simple, basic movements that should be performed one after the other. In other words, just keep moving for the recommended time and you will get all the benefits of aerobics. Some of the warm up, aerobic, and cool-down exercises are similar to the ones performed on the trampoline. Make exercise fun by listening to your favorite music while you move.

SAMPLE FLOOR AEROBICS PROGRAM

WEEKS 1 TO 3

3x per week: **Monday/Wednesday/Friday or**
Tuesday/Thursday/Saturday or Sunday

WARM UP:

Begin by leading with the right leg.

March in place	1 minute
Toe Taps	2 minutes
Runner's Lunge	hold the stretch 10 seconds
Calf Raises	8x
Hamstring Stretch	hold 10 seconds
Back Stretch	hold 10 seconds

Repeat the warm up exercise sequence with the left leg leading the movement.

TOTAL TIME 9 MINUTES

Check and record your pulse and glucose, and exertion rating. Drink 6 oz of water.

AEROBICS:

Continue stepping in place, pumping your arms as you step. Lift your feet about 2 to 3 inches. Gradually progress to a light jog, increasing the range of motion of your legs and arms. After 5 minutes, perform the following arm movements for one minute each.

Front Raise	Biceps Curl
Side Raise	Low Rows
Front Crisscross	Pullbacks
Overhead Press	Pulldowns
Front Press	Tricep Press

Continuing to jog, check your pulse and glucose, and record your exertion level. Drink 6 oz of water. Then perform the following floor aerobics exercises for 1 minute each.

Low Skip Kicks	Knee Lifts
Jump Rope	Knee Pump
Jump Rope Wide	Hamstring Curls
Jump Rope Narrow/Wide	Jab-Bob and Weave
Half Jacks	V-Step
Tap Backs	

TOTAL TIME APPROXIMATELY 26 MINUTES

COOL-DOWN:

Step Touches on the floor	2 minutes
Runner's Lunge	
right leg	hold 20 seconds
left leg	hold 20 seconds
Hamstring Stretch	
right leg	hold 20 seconds
left leg	hold 20 seconds
Back Stretch	hold 10 seconds, release the stretch, and repeat
Shoulder Stretch	
right shoulder	hold 20 seconds
left shoulder	hold 20 seconds
Chest Stretch	20 seconds

TOTAL TIME APPROXIMATELY 6 MINUTES

TOTAL EXERCISE SESSION TIME APPROXIMATELY 41 MINUTES

Check and record your pulse and glucose, and exertion rating. Drink 6 oz of water.

WEEKS 4 TO 6

3x per week: **Monday/Wednesday/Friday or**
Tuesday/Thursday/Saturday or Sunday

WARM UP:

Begin by leading with the right leg.

March in place	2 minutes
Toe Taps	2 minutes
Runner's Lunge	hold the stretch 10 seconds
Calf Raises	8x
Hamstring Stretch	hold 10 seconds
Back Stretch	hold 10 seconds

Repeat the warm up exercise sequence with the left leg leading the movement.

TOTAL TIME 12 MINUTES

Check and record your pulse and glucose, and exertion rating. Drink 6 oz of water.

AEROBICS:

Continue stepping in place, pumping your arms as you step. Lift your feet about 2 to 3 inches. Gradually progress to a light jog, increasing the range of motion of your legs and arms. After 5 minutes, perform the following arm movements for 1 1/2 minutes each.

Front Raise	Biceps Curl
Side Raise	Low Rows
Front Crisscross	Pullbacks
Overhead Press	Pulldowns
Front Press	Tricep Press

Continuing to jog, check your pulse and glucose, and record your exertion level. Drink 6 oz of water. Then perform the following floor aerobics exercises for 1 minute each.

Low Skip Kicks	Knee Lifts
Jump Rope	Knee Pump
Jump Rope Wide	Hamstring Curls
Jump Rope Narrow/Wide	Jab-Bob and Weave
Half Jacks	V-Step
Tap Backs	

TOTAL TIME APPROXIMATELY 31 MINUTES

COOL-DOWN:

Step Touches on the floor	2 minutes
Runner's Lunge	
right leg	hold 20 seconds
left leg	hold 20 seconds
Hamstring Stretch	
right leg	hold 20 seconds
left leg	hold 20 seconds
Back Stretch	hold 10 seconds, release the stretch, and repeat
Shoulder Stretch	
right shoulder	hold 20 seconds
left shoulder	hold 20 seconds
Chest Stretch	20 seconds

TOTAL TIME APPROXIMATELY 6 MINUTES

TOTAL EXERCISE SESSION TIME APPROXIMATELY 49 MINUTES

Check and record your pulse and glucose, and exertion rating. Drink 6 oz of water.

WEEKS 7 TO 9

3x per week: Monday/Wednesday/Friday or

Tuesday/Thursday/Saturday or Sunday

WARM UP:

Begin by leading with the right leg.

March in place	2 minutes
Toe Taps	2 minutes
Runner's Lunge	hold the stretch 10 seconds
Calf Raises	8x
Hamstring Stretch	hold 10 seconds
Back Stretch	hold 10 seconds

Repeat the warm up exercise sequence with the left leg leading the movement.

TOTAL TIME 12 MINUTES

Check and record your pulse and glucose, and exertion rating. Drink 6 oz of water.

AEROBICS:

Continue stepping in place, pumping your arms as you step. Lift your feet about 2 to 3 inches. Gradually progress to a light jog, increasing the range of motion of your legs and arms. After 5 minutes, perform the following arm movements for one and a half minutes each.

Front Raise	Biceps Curl
Side Raise	Low Rows
Front Crisscross	Pullbacks
Overhead Press	Pulldowns
Front Press	Tricep Press

Continuing to jog, check your pulse and glucose, and record your exertion level. Drink 6 oz of water. Then perform the following floor aerobics exercises for 1 minute each.

Low Skip Kicks	Knee Lifts
Jump Rope	Knee Pump
Jump Rope Wide	Hamstring Curls
Jump Rope Narrow/Wide	Jab-Bob and Weave
Half Jacks	V-Step
Tap Backs	

TOTAL TIME APPROXIMATELY 36 MINUTES

COOL-DOWN:

Step Touches on the floor	2 minutes
Runner's Lunge	
right leg	hold 30 seconds
left leg	hold 30 seconds
Hamstring Stretch	
right leg	hold 30 seconds
left leg	hold 30 seconds
Back Stretch	hold 20 seconds, release the stretch, and repeat
Shoulder Stretch	
right shoulder	hold 30 seconds
left shoulder	hold 30 seconds
Chest Stretch	30 seconds

TOTAL TIME APPROXIMATELY 8 MINUTES

TOTAL EXERCISE SESSION TIME APPROXIMATELY 56 MINUTES

Check and record your pulse and glucose, and exertion rating. Drink 6 oz of water.

WEEKS 10+

Follow the program from Weeks 7 to 9 but add an extra day of training per week. For example:

Monday/Wednesday/Friday/Saturday or Sunday

Tuesday/Thursday/Saturday/Sunday

In addition to the programs offered so far, a walking program or exercise on a stationary cycle are excellent methods of aerobic conditioning for the diabetic. On the days you don't use the mini-trampoline or do floor aerobics, you can take a walk or cycle. Or perhaps you would like to go for a walk and just do a portion of the mini-trampoline. Customize the program to meet your needs and what feels right for your body.

14

The Strength-Training Program

Start with the warm up movements on pages 143 to 148. Then per-form all of the strength-training exercises from Chapter 10 according to the following program. Cool-down by following the stretches given in the flexibility section on pages 130 to 141.

A Sample Strength Training Program

Week 1 to 2

Repetitions:	8x each exercise
Resistance:	3 to 5 lbs
Set:	1
Frequency:	2 nonconsecutive days

Weeks 3 to 4

Repetitions:	10x each exercise
Resistance:	3 to 5 lbs
Set:	1
Frequency:	2 nonconsecutive days

Weeks 5 to 6

Repetitions:	12 to 15x each exercise
Resistance:	3 to 5 lbs
Set:	1
Frequency:	2 nonconsecutive days

Weeks 7 to 8

Repetitions:	8x each exercise
Resistance:	5 to 8 lbs
Set:	1
Frequency:	2 nonconsecutive days

Weeks 9 to 10

Repetitions:	10x each exercise
Resistance:	5 to 8 lbs
Set:	1
Frequency:	2 nonconsecutive days

Weeks 11 to 12

Repetitions:	12 to 15x each exercise
Resistance:	5 to 8 lbs
Set:	2
Frequency:	2 nonconsecutive days

At this point you should determine how to best intensify your strength program. You can add an extra day or another set, or increase the weight. However, the recommendation for diabetics is moderate resistance and not heavy weight lifting.

15

Fitness Walking

Fitness walking is different from regular walking in that you must pay attention to the position of your arms, torso, and legs as you walk. There is a greater conscious effort to use the leg and arm muscles to make it an effective workout. The length of your stride and the range of motion of your arms play a part in distinguishing fitness walking from regular walking. Walking is the most universally recommended activity. You can't beat it! It doesn't cost anything and you don't need any special equipment. It's convenient and a safe form of exercise for diabetics. You do need to follow the same rules as with any other form of aerobic training. It must be of sufficient intensity and duration to make it effective for weight loss and health benefits. You really need to use those leg and arm muscles to add power to your walk and elevate your heart rate to make fitness walking work.

The speed at which you walk should be brisk to make it effective. If this is not possible at first, than do what you can to increase your pace to a brisk to fast walk. Below is a breakdown of how fast you should walk and how to increase your speed as you become more fit. This is just a guideline; if you need to start at a slower, more comfortable speed, that's OK. The important thing is that you are moving, and over time you can increase the pace. In order for the program to be effective you will need to walk long enough each day, so I will give you guidelines for duration as well.

Walking Speed

Weeks 1 to 3
quick: 3.5 mph (17 minutes per mile) - 20 minutes

Weeks 4 to 7
brisk: 4 mph (15 minutes per mile) - 25 minutes

Weeks 8 to 10
brisk: 4 mph (15 minutes per mile) - 30 minutes

Weeks 11 to 13
fast: 4.6 mph (13 minutes per mile) - 35 minutes

Each week thereafter increase the time by 5 minutes until you are walking for 40 to 45 minutes.

Use the warm ups and cool-downs given in this book at the beginning and end of your fitness walk. Follow the same guidelines for hydration, monitoring the intensity of the workout, and monitoring glucose levels. You should wear a hip pack containing a glucose monitor, a carbohydrate, and a pen and piece of paper to record your exertion rating, heart rate, and glucose levels.

Walking technique is the next critical element in fitness walking. The goal is to use the large muscles in the legs to burn more calories and make walking more aerobic. The more intensely we use our muscles, the more oxygen we use and the more calories we burn.

Walking Technique

Your posture should be straight and tall. Lift your ribcage away from your pelvis. Your eyes should be focused forward in a straight line. Open up your stride by reaching out with your stride (front) leg from the hip when you step out. As the leg comes forward your heel should strike the ground first, and then your foot should roll, with your toes hitting the ground last. Push off with the ball of the foot as you bring your back leg forward to add power to your stride. The exchange that occurs with the right and left legs, reaching forward with each step, should be fluid and smooth. Your feet should be parallel, your steps almost one behind the other. To practice your walking technique, draw a chalk line on the pavement. The insides of your feet should follow along the path of the line.

Aim for a long stride as this will keep it smooth and not choppy. Your arms should be bent at a 90-degree angles throughout your workout. Let the arms pump front to back in a straight line. Your body weight should be centered between your legs. Do not lean forward or backward and relax into your stride. Do not place a lot of tension in your body, but do try to use a full range of motion when you walk.

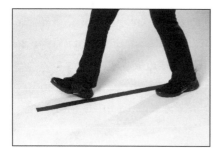 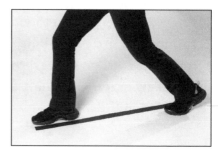

16

Cycling

Cycling, whether on a stationary bike or on the road, is a great non-weight-bearing exercise. For diabetics with peripheral neuropathy, it is ideal. It places minimal stress on the joints, and a bicycle is an easy piece of equipment to operate. But there are a few things you should know.

Proper Bike Fit

You need to make adjustments to the seat height to minimize stress to your knees and to make biking more comfortable. When you stand next to the bike, the seat should be at hip height. Next, sit on the seat and place your feet on the pedals. Pedal slowly. When you straighten out your leg at the point where the pedal is straight down and closest to the floor, your knee should be bent slightly (5-degrees). Any more or less and adjustments should be made.

Form and Technique

Keep your head up and eyes focused forward. Your shoulders should be down and relaxed. Do not lock your elbows or lean on your arms. Keep your elbows soft and wrists straight, and your spine and hips in a neutral alignment. As you pedal keep your feet flat, as if you were swiping or brushing them along the floor. Don't pedal with your toes pointing down.

Intensity and Duration

You need to follow the same guidelines and suggestions given for other methods of aerobic training. Always begin with a warm up. When cycling, you can warm up by pedaling for 10 minutes at no resistance. Increase the resistance after the warm up to a comfortable level and maintain that resistance for 20 minutes. Cool-down by pedaling with no resistance for 5 minutes. End your cycling session with the stretches featured in this book.

A Sample Cycling Program

weeks 1 to 3
20 minutes,
light to moderate resistance
3 to 5x per week

week 4
25 minutes
light to moderate resistance
3 to 5x per week

week 5
30 minutes
light to moderate resistance
4 to 5x per week

week 6
30 minutes
moderate intensity
4 to 5x per week

week 7
35 minutes
moderate intensity
4 to 5x per week

week 8
40 minutes
moderate intensity
5+ x per week

Appendix A

Training Log

Day: _____

Date: _____

Time: _____

TYPE OF EXERCISE

Aerobic: _____

Duration: _____

Intensity: heart rate_____   perceived exertion_____

Glucose Levels: pre-exercise_____ during exercise_____ postexercise_____

STRENGTH

Exercises Performed:

Overhead Press:

	weight_____	# reps_____	# sets_____
Lateral Raise:	weight_____	# reps_____	# sets_____
Front Raise:	weight_____	# reps_____	# sets_____
Pullbacks:	weight_____	# reps_____	# sets_____
Biceps Curls:	weight_____	# reps_____	# sets_____
Squats:		# reps_____	# sets_____
Hip Hiker:		# reps_____	# sets_____
Chest Press:	weight_____	# reps_____	# sets_____
Flies:	weight_____	# reps_____	# sets_____

Triceps Extensions:

weight_____   # reps_____   # sets_____

Crossover Triceps Extensions:

weight_____   # reps_____   # sets_____

Curl-Ups: # reps_____   # sets_____

Core Stabilization:

reps_____   # sets_____

Crossover Crunch:

weight_____   # reps_____   # sets_____

Side Leg Lifts: # reps_____   # sets_____

Inner Thigh Lifts: # reps_____   # sets_____

Back Leg Lifts: # reps_____   # sets_____

Modified Push-Ups:

reps_____   # sets_____

Shoulder Extensions:

weight_____   # reps_____   # sets_____

Glucose Levels: pre-exercise_____ during exercise_____ postexercise_____

Flexibility:

 # Exercises Performed _____

Medication: Type_____ Dose_____ Time_____

Pre-exercise Meals: Time_____ Type_____

Hydration: Fluid Type_____ Amount_____

Appendix B

Websites

American Diabetes Association

www.diabetes.org

Centers for Disease Control and Prevention

www.cdc.gov/diabetes

National Diabetes Education Program

www.ndep.nih.gov

National Diabetes Information Clearinghouse

www.niddk.nih.gov

Appendix C

References

Caffrey, R.M. "Diabetes Under Control: Are All Syringes Created Equal?" *American Journal of Nursing*, June 2003, pp. 46 49.

ACSM's* Resource Manual for Guidelines for Exercise Testing and Prescription. (1998) Williams and Wilkins.

Thomassian, B.D. "Type 2 Diabetes Among Youth Reaches Epidemic Proportions." *Nursing Spectrum*, November 2004.

Sherman, W., and Albright, A. "Exercise and Type 1 Diabetes." *Sports Science Exchange.* May 1990.

Sherman, W., and Albright, A. "Exercise and Type 2 Diabetes." *Sports Science Exchange.* March 1992.

Colberg, S.R. "Exercise: A Diabetics 'Cure' For Many?" *ACSM's* Health & Fitness Journal* March/April 2001.

**American College of Sports Medicine*